The Psychophysiology of Low Back Pain

Nicola Adams BSc (Hons) PhD MCSP
Senior Lecturer, School of Health and Social Sciences,
Coventry University, Coventry, UK

Contributions by
Douglas N Taylor PhD
Director, Centre for Behavioural Medicine,
New York, USA

Michael J Rose PhD SRP MCSP
Programme Co ordinator,
Wirral Low Back Pain Rehabilitation Programme,
Wirral Hospital NHS Trust, Wirral, UK

Foreword by
John Ravey PhD
Lecturer School of Behavioural and Communication Sciences,
University of Ulster, Jordanstown, UK

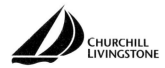

CHURCHILL
LIVINGSTONE

NEW YORK EDINBURGH LONDON MADRID MELBOURNE SAN FRANCISCO TOKYO 1997

CHURCHILL LIVINGSTONE
Medical Division of Pearson Professional Limited

Distributed in the United States of America by Churchill Livingstone,
650 Avenue of the Americas, New York, N.Y. 10011, and by associated
companies, branches and representatives throughout the world.

© Pearson Professional Limited 1997

First published 1997

ISBN 0 443 05259 X

British Library Cataloguing in Publication Data
A catalogue record for this book is available from the British Library.

Library of Congress Cataloging in Publication Data
A catalog record for this book is available from the Library of Congress.

The
publisher's
policy is to use
**paper manufactured
from sustainable forests**

Printed by Longman Singapore Publishers (Pte) Ltd
Printed in Singapore

Contents

Foreword

For all the happiness mankind can gain
Is not in pleasure, but in rest from pain
John Dryden (1631–1700)

The effort to find ways of alleviating human pain has a history as long as the history of therapy itself and is, in many ways, central to the practice of medicine. There has been an explosion of information and knowledge about pain during the second half of the twentieth century and this has led to increasingly complex theoretical models which can no longer be thought of as being the property of any one branch of science. Society has also become considerably more complex during the same period and the social and economic consequences of pain, especially chronic pain, have been increasingly recognised. With the wide range of professions involved in the study and treatment of low back pain, it is becoming more and more difficult for the individual practitioner to keep track of the information available.

This book brings together a number of the strands. While it is wide ranging, it is no shallow review. It concentrates in depth on a number of related topics and their interactions in a way that not only reflects current theoretical interests and scientific research in several disciplines, but which also is of practical use to the clinician. The neurophysiological bases of pain are recognised and examined in detail as are biochemical factors which influence the experience of pain. Such biological correlates of chronic pain are, however, seen as inadequate in themselves as a description of the individual's experience of pain. The author gives equal weight to psychological and psychosocial influences while avoiding doctrinaire adherence to any one theoretical stance. Ultimately, the focus is on the patient, with chapters dealing with the assessment and alternative approaches to treatment to suit the needs of the individual. As a graduate practitioner with clinical experience at both pre-doctoral and post-doctoral level, Dr Adams has published much of her own research on many of the topics dealt with in this book. She is a member of several professional national and international organisations including the British Psychological Society, the Chartered Society of Physiotherapy, the International Association for the Study of Pain and the Association for Applied Psychophysiology and Biofeedback (USA). The scope of the book reflects her background of rigorous academic research and practical expertise and it should make available those assets to members of the great variety of disciplines which now seek to give mankind *rest from pain*.

J.R.

Preface

Despite the great technological advances that have been made in science and medicine, the prevalent conditions of the common cold and low back pain (LBP) still evade a rapid intervention strategy for recovery. While the common cold runs its course, LBP in a significant number of cases does not resolve and progresses to a chronic pain syndrome. LBP causes much suffering, distress and incapacitation to the individual and has great economic significance in terms of lost output and disability payments (Klaber-Moffett et al 1995).

For each individual the pain experience is different, due not only to physiological characteristics but also to psychosocial factors. Biomechanical problems affect the spine, but factors such as depression, anxiety and emotional distress affect the CNS control of posture and movement with resultant physiological symptoms such as muscle dysfunction and disorders of posture and gait. Therefore, although physical impairment may be ameliorated by physical intervention, it is also necessary to address psychological factors for maximal response to intervention strategies. Thus, the complex nature of the condition means that a range of professions are involved in the study and treatment of LBP, each lending their own particular expertise to the condition. Recently combined treatment approaches have pooled this expertise and have demonstrated considerable success in the management of these patients.

This book reviews the physiological (biomechanical), neurochemical and psychological components of LBP. The latter are reviewed in detail; their interaction to produce the experience of pain is presented and the way in which treatment strategies may intervene and modulate the experience of pain is discussed. This serves as a physiological basis for the use of psychological principles to augment physical treatment.

No one theoretical stance has been adopted and theories from several disciplines and schools of thought have been drawn together. As such, the text is written for the range of professionals who are treating LBP, irrespective of their discipline, in order that they may combine assessment and management procedures presented in this text to augment their practice.

Many patients with chronic low back pain report, in addition to their pain, many diverse symptoms such as fatigue, gastrointestinal disturbances, poor peripheral circulation, general aches and pains, low energy and feeling 'down'. To understand and correctly interpret these symptoms, it is important to understand the processes involved in the production of pain. Chapters 2 and 3 detail the neurophysiological and neurochemical processes involved in pain so that the practitioner is able to distinguish between symptoms due to physiological and neurochemical responses to pain and factors such as abnormal illness behaviour. Assessment procedures are detailed in Chapter 7, and Chapter 8 reviews the psychological principles and techniques used in the treatment of pain.

My own research has been concerned with the investigation of the components of back pain in an attempt to determine their interaction to produce the pain experience. This book has been written from studies, published literature and clinical experience. It does not purport to have an answer to all cases. However, my belief is that accurate diagnosis is essential, as is early intervention and appropriate consideration to the psychological factors involved in pain.

No interaction is as important as that between patient and practitioner, and the final chapter is devoted to this topic. Many patients with similar signs and symptoms may respond favourably to different treatment approaches implemented by different practitioners. Several studies have suggested that it is not only the physical treatment that is advocated but, equally importantly, the psychological qualities of the patient–practitioner relationship can be major mediators for improvement. Thus the practitioner has considerable power to define outcomes of treatment.

This book is written for the professionals who treat LBP patients and ultimately for the individuals who suffer from this distressing complaint.

Coventry 1997

N.A.

Acknowledgements

I am grateful to many people who contributed directly and indirectly to this text.

I would first like to thank my contributing authors, Dr Douglas Taylor and Dr Michael Rose for giving their time and expertise to produce the material and the staff at Churchill Livingstone for their guidance and support during the process of writing this text.

I would like to thank my family, brothers and sisters-in-law, Jonathan, Seana, Tristan and Lorraine and my friends, many of whom I regard as family, for their unconditional love and support.

I am especially grateful to Dr John Ravey and Professor Jean Bell for their unfailing and inspirational guidance, support and encouragement, both personally and professionally, over many years. I would also like to thank Dorothy Whittington for her encouragement and direction to embark on this text.

I owe a debt of great personal gratitude to Dr Milliken and Professor Atkinson for their medical expertise and for caring.

1

Introduction

Nicola Adams

INTRODUCTION AND EPIDEMIOLOGY

The experience of pain is a subjective event which is influenced not only by anatomical, physiological and biochemical factors in response to tissue damage, but also by a number of psychological and social factors. The importance of psychological and social factors in the perception and response to pain has been increasingly recognised, particularly in the area of chronic low back pain (LBP). This growing awareness has led to a gradual progression from treatment to alleviate physical symptoms to educating patients to manage their pain. Often such approaches are based on psychological principles and approaches which augment physical or pharmacological intervention.

The behaviour of those with similar painful disorders may differ considerably because of differences in psychological characteristics and social circumstances and different response patterns to pain and impairment of function. These different patterns of behaviour should be considered in the diagnosis and management of painful conditions.

This is of particular relevance in low back pain as it is a major cause of morbidity, disability, limitation of activity and economic loss. Most studies have found that 60–80% of the population are affected with LBP at some time during their lives (Frymoyer et al 1983). In the UK it is estimated that the costs of back pain to the NHS probably lie between £265–383 million per annum (Klaber–Moffett et al 1995).

Lumbar impairments most frequently cause activity limitation among persons under 45 years in the US. They rank third after heart disease and arthritis in persons aged 45–64 years. Nevertheless most episodes of low back pain do not seriously incapacitate people. Among those LBP patients consulting general practitioners, almost 90% improve within 1–3 months, regardless of treatment (Dixon 1973). About 7% of persons developing low back pain report still having pain after 6 months (Horal 1969, Vukmir 1991) and it is primarily these people who are responsible for the high costs of low back pain. Frequently, persons absent from work due to back pain do not demonstrate any objective signs on physical examination (Vallfors 1985). In the absence of clear organic pathology, there are often a number of psychological factors which are contributing to the pain experience.

Such psychological factors contributing to pain and their psychophysiological mediation are discussed in this book.

NATURE OF THE PAIN EXPERIENCE

In addition to the experience of pain, an individual may also manifest psychological, autonomic and neuroendocrine responses, such as fatigue, gastrointestinal upsets, feeling down or depressed, and avoid physical and social activity. Many systems are affected by the experience of pain and, as pain is influenced by physiological and biomechanical factors, psychological factors and immunological and neuroendocrinological factors, these diverse symptoms are unsurprising. These systems are frequently interrelated and affecting one often affects the other. Thus psychological and physiological factors are closely interrelated. All pain is felt in the mind, however mediated, and for the purposes of this text, the effect of psychological factors on other systems and ultimately the overall experience and response to pain will be presented.

Thus a model of LBP is presented incorporating psychological, physiological and biochemical components (Fig. 1.1). Each component affects the other and thus it is possible to intervene at each level to affect outcome. Whatever the treatment approach assumed, it is possible to incorporate a psychological approach that augments the treatment.

In order to understand the pain experience, it is necessary to understand the physiological, biochemical and psychological mechanisms involved at spinal and central levels.

In the following chapters, these mechanisms and their interactions are presented.

Interaction of psychological, biomechanical and biochemical factors

The aspects involved in the pathogenesis of low back pain have been reported to be emotional factors such as depression and anxiety (Krishnan et al 1985, French 1989, Klaber-Moffett & Richardson 1995) and biomechanical factors such as changes in soft tissues, facet joints and inter-

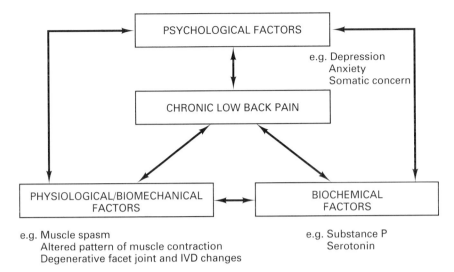

Figure 1.1   A three-factor model of low back pain.

vertebral disc (IVD). There are also biochemical events at the stages involved in the pathology of back pain, e.g. at an area of tissue trauma there is release of endogenous chemicals such as serotonin (5HT), prostaglandins and substance P into the extracellular fluid (ECF) that surrounds the nociceptors. Not only do these chemicals have a direct action on nociception but they also have an indirect action on the local microcirculation resulting in symptoms such as temperature changes in the affected area and other autonomic effects. Somatovisceral reactions may also occur and in addition there may be effects on mood and sleep (Cesselin et al 1993). Thus diverse symptoms may be experienced at an early stage. In most cases, resolution occurs within 3 months. A small percentage of patients progress to a chronic pain syndrome where pain report and resultant disability exceed peripheral input. In the absence of discriminative biomechanical factors, it is suggested that other factors, perhaps psychological or biochemical, singly or in combination, may generate and perpetuate an abnormal neural circuitry with concomitant depressive symptoms, and autonomic and neuroendocrine responses. There are a number of significant psychological factors in LBP, including depression. These factors are reviewed in Chapters 5 and 6. However, it is debated whether depressive symptoms are the cause of LBP or its result (Polatin et al 1993).

It is difficult to ascertain to what extent biochemical factors affect psychological factors and vice versa. Physiological/biomechanical factors are certainly contributory and are more straightforward. With prolonged inactivity, pathology increases to involve other structures, with resultant

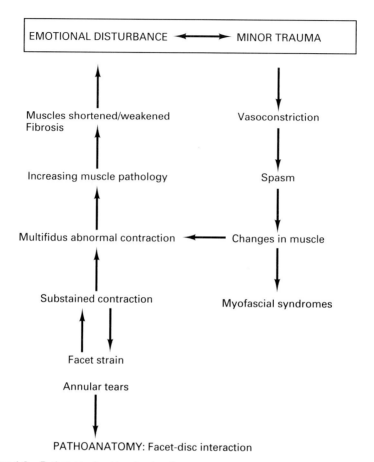

Figure 1.2 Pathogenesis of low back pain.

loss of function and increase in pain. At this stage, patients often report feelings of frustration and depression as they perceive a loss of control and an increase in feelings of hopelessness about their condition.

Thus a cycle is generated and maintained (Fig. 1.2), and treatment should aim at interrupting this cycle. Different treatments aim to interrupt the cycle at different points, and therefore the potential for these patients to respond to a wide variety of interventions is great.

Definitions of pain

Although the effect of psychological factors on pain has been mentioned, before examining these in more detail, it is necessary to understand more about what pain is, in order to understand how it may be influenced. Merskey & Spear (1967) defined pain as:

an unpleasant sensory and emotional experience associated with actual or potential tissue damage or described in terms of such damage.

It is a personal experience and is composed of both physical and psychological factors. It is a specific sensation brought about by damage or threat of damage; therefore it has a high subjective content as to the individual's interpretation of 'threat of damage'. Like any other sensory stimulus, pain has a threshold, i.e. noxious stimulation must reach a certain intensity before pain is felt. This is known as the pain perception threshold (PPT) and is defined as:

The least intensity of noxious stimulation at which a subject consciously perceives pain (Wells et al 1988).

The PPT is relatively constant from person to person. It is the pain tolerance threshold (PTT) that is highly variable from person to person and is affected by psychological and emotional factors. The PTT is defined by Wells et al (1988) as:

The greatest intensity of noxious stimulation an individual can bear.

When pain goes beyond a person's tolerance level, then the person will seek help. Acute pain may be of survival value and therefore beneficial in that it calls attention to a real or perceived threat. It is frequently a symptom of underlying disease (Echternach 1987). Chronic pain on the other hand, appears to have no such value and seems to comprise peripheral input and changes in neural functioning which sustain pain circuitry beyond peripheral input. Echternach (1987) and Wu & Smith (1987) suggested that chronic pain may be a disease on its own and not simply an extension of acute pain.

Interpretation of pain

The experience of pain represents an individual's interpretation of the intensity of a particular stimulus, as well as an assessment of whether or not it constitutes a significant threat to well-being. These judgements are made at cortical level, but several subcortical structures play an important role in determining the reaction of the individual. Cutaneous and visceral receptors, peripheral nerve fibres and CNS pathways constitute a transmission system which functions in the modulation and conduction of impulses to higher levels (Melzack & Wall 1989). Receptors and pathways are concerned with relaying impulses originating from the application of the noxious stimuli. A particular stimulus may be perceived as painful depending on a number of highly variable factors. These factors can be physical, psychological or emotional, and singly or in combination may significantly influence perception of a stimulus (Echternach 1987).

It can therefore be seen that pain is often a necessary warning and protective experience to prevent further noxious harm. It is also of value in that it sets limits on activity and enforces inactivity that is often important for recovery. However, beyond this, pain can rapidly become a self-sustaining abnormal noxious agent in its own right, causing functional disability and psychosocial strain (Bengston 1983).

Differences between acute and chronic pain

As stated previously, acute pain is finite in nature. An episode of low back pain usually resolves within 4–12 weeks. If pain persists beyond 6 months, it is then classified as chronic. Unlike acute pain which serves as a protective mechanism, chronic pain does not appear to serve any purpose. There are also different features of acute and chronic pain. Acute pain tends to be sharp and localised, whereas chronic pain tends to be dull and diffuse in nature. Chronic pain sufferers tend to experience many diverse symptoms and there are a number of psychological and behavioural factors that are involved in the experience of chronic pain. These are presented in later chapters.

In addition, acute pain tends to respond well to treatment, whereas chronic pain is more difficult to treat. Chronic pain also has a tendency to recur, suggesting perpetuating psychological and neurophysiological involvement.

RISK FACTORS

There are a number of characteristics that may contribute to LBP. These include:

Demographic characteristics

First episodes of low back pain occur most often between the ages of 20 and 40 years (Bigos et al 1986). Males and females report low back pain with approximately equal frequency, though work-related injuries for which compensation is received are more common in men (Snook 1982).

Low back pain is more often reported by those in lower socioeconomic classes and this is probably attributable to the higher proportion of people in these classes who work in manual labour. A number of risk factors have been identified in developing low back pain. These include occupational risk factors such as heavy manual work and sedentary work and driving.

Heavy manual work

Low back pain is more common in heavy manual workers than in other workers (Walsh et al 1989). The occupations with the highest rate of back injuries and absence from work attributable to back pain are truck drivers and ambulance drivers. Most injuries occur in association with the loading and unloading of trucks or when lifting immobile patients in awkward and biomechanically disadvantaged positions and lifting stretchers into ambulances (Gamble et al 1991). These groups are followed by material handlers, nurses and auxiliary nurses who may be lifting heavy immobile weights such as anaesthetised patients or hemiplegic patients. It appears that jobs requiring frequent lifting of objects weighing 25 lb or more are associated with an increase in risk, while lifting lighter objects is not associated with an increased risk (Andersson 1981). In addition, sudden maximal effort appears to be associated with low back pain, and frequent stretching, reaching, pulling and pushing may also be risk factors (Damkot et al 1984). This is common in both ambulance drivers and policemen, as both jobs are characterised by long periods of relative inactivity and sudden heavy and occasionally violent activity

Sedentary work and driving

Some evidence suggests that jobs that are primarily sedentary increase the risk for low back pain. Since intradiscal pressure is higher in the sitting position than when standing or lying supine, it is possible that there is an increased risk in sedentary occupations. In addition, these people may have less opportunity to move around and may develop muscle strain as a result of maintained postures, contributing to pain. Secretaries and clerical workers frequently complain of upper or lower back pain due to maintained sedentary postures (Kelsey et al 1992).

Fitness and muscle strength

Some studies have suggested that back and abdominal muscle strength may protect against back injuries, as strong muscles may alleviate part of the mechanical stresses on the spine. Findings have been inconclusive and it has been suggested that back pain also leads to muscle weakness; therefore this weakness may be the result of back pain rather than its cause (Asfour & Ayoub 1984).

Medical history

Previous back pain is an important risk factor in developing future episodes of pain. Possible mechanisms may include loss of extensibility of normal tissue due to the formation of scar tissue from a previously healed injury. This causes loss of spinal mobility, so if a movement occurs further than the available range, pain will occur. Another predisposing factor is weakness of the spinal musculature due to avoidance of activity. A final possible mechanism is that neurochemical changes may cause alterations in motor activity and muscle function which may predispose to recurrence (Bombardier et al 1994).

Smoking

Several studies show an association between cigarette smoking and low back pain. Current smokers have about twice the risk for prolapsed lumbar disc as non-smokers, while the risk among those who have given up smoking for more than 1 year is similar to the risk in those who have never smoked. Possible mechanisms for the association between back pain and smoking include reduced oxygenation of the lumbar discs and inhibition of fibrinolytic activity (Meade et al 1979).

Pregnancy

Back pain in the late stages of pregnancy is relatively common due to the exaggerated lordosis in the lumbar spine. Other physiological mechanisms include changes in body water content, endocrine changes, and engorgement of epidural veins (MacEvilly & Buggy 1996). Hormonal changes at childbirth may cause laxity of the sacroiliac ligaments to allow for the birth of the baby and some mothers experience sacroiliac pain after birth. This may be associated with bending, reaching, and lifting the baby. In addition, epidural analgesia may also cause some local pain. For a fuller discussion the reader is referred to MacEvilly and Buggy 1996.

Psychological and sociological factors

Psychological factors are important in both the perception and response to pain, whereas sociological factors such as the nature of a person's occupation, or financial implications may have a profound effect on the severity and extent of disruption of back pain. For example, it may not be as easy for an unskilled manual worker to move to another occupation. These sociological factors may also lead to psychological stress, which may also exacerbate the condition.

Various psychosocial factors have been implicated in low back pain. These include personality characteristics such as depression and anxiety, beliefs about pain, patterns of illness behaviour and social and work environment.

These factors should be taken into consideration when the practitioner is examining a patient with low back pain. Accurate assessment and diagnosis is of vital importance and this is presented in Chapter 7. The nature of the patient–practitioner relationship may also influence the outcomes of treatment irrespective of the treatment advocated by the particular professional background of the clinician.

TREATMENT FOR LOW BACK PAIN ˙

Conservative treatment for LBP has traditionally been rest, analgesia and physical therapy such as mobilisation, manipulation and electrotherapy (Koes et al 1991, Dimaggio & Mooney 1987). A critical review of published literature of these approaches may be found in Klaber–Moffett et al 1995.

Treatment has become multimodal and increasingly multidisciplinary, in recognition of the number of factors involved in the aetiology and perpetuation of LBP, in particular chronic LBP. Irrespective of the particular discipline in which the practitioner has trained, it is necessary to address psychological aspects of the pain experience. Addressing these factors has been shown to be effective in management programmes. Anecdotally, any practitioner who specialises in the physical treatment of back pain, acknowledges the role of psychological factors such as anxiety, loss of earnings, inability to cope, etc., and often intuitively reassures, educates and sets goals for the patient to achieve in addition to the physical treatment. The interaction between patient and practitioner has been shown to be a significant mediator for improvement and this is further discussed in Chapter 9.

Each discipline thus provides a unique contribution to the management of low back pain, and disciplines can be seen to be intervening at different levels to affect outcome. Detailed assessment thus provides an indication of the extent of physiological/biomechanical and psychological signs and symptoms in the individual patient, in order that appropriate treatment may be implemented.

PURPOSE OF THIS TEXT

The purpose of this text is to enhance understanding of the interaction of factors involved in low back pain and to suggest ways of expanding, or indeed merely reinforcing, existing practices.

In order to do this, the neurophysiological, biochemical and psychological aspects of pain are presented and then the ways in which the practitioner may assess and modulate the pain experience are addressed.

2

Neurophysiological factors in low back pain

Nicola Adams

INTRODUCTION

This chapter details the neuroanatomical and neurophysiological sub-strates involved in the production of the experience of low back pain.

The processes involved in the production and response to pain are shown in Figure 2.1.

PERIPHERAL SUBSTRATES

Sensory receptors

A sensory stimulus is detected and then transduced into a code of electri-cal nerve impulses by a sensory receptor; afferent nerves then transmit the impulses from the receptor to the brain and spinal cord (Stein 1982). Different types of sensory receptor exist for the appreciation of different stimuli. A receptor may in general terms be defined as a structure, usually a nerve ending, which converts some specific form of energy into nervous impulses (Bowsher 1988). Sensory receptors are found in the covering layers of the body, special sense organs, muscles and joints, etc. Nociceptors are receptors that respond to noxious stimuli only. The lumbosacral nociceptor receptor systems are found in skin, subcutaneous and adipose

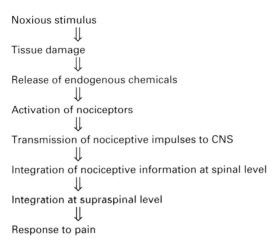

Noxious stimulus
⇓
Tissue damage
⇓
Release of endogenous chemicals
⇓
Activation of nociceptors
⇓
Transmission of nociceptive impulses to CNS
⇓
Integration of nociceptive information at spinal level
⇓
Integration at supraspinal level
⇓
Response to pain

Figure 2.1   Processes involved in the production of pain.

tissue, capsule of the facet and sacroiliac joints, ligaments, dura mater and walls of the intramuscular arteries within the lumbosacral muscles (Burgess & Perl 1973, Jayson 1987).

Polymodal C fibre nociceptors

The polymodal C fibre nociceptors (sometimes referred to as 'free nerve endings') are found in the deeper part of the skin and in virtually every other tissue except the nervous system itself. They are frequently sensitive to mechanical, thermal and chemical noxious stimuli (Wells et al 1988).

A-delta nociceptors

The A-delta nociceptors are distributed fairly superficially on the skin. Small numbers are also found in joints and muscle. The majority are sensitive only to high-intensity mechanical stimuli and a small number are also sensitive to noxious temperature changes (Wells et al 1988).

Nerve fibres

Nerve fibres are classified according to their diameter and conduction velocity. They are illustrated in Table 2.1.

Specialized cutaneous receptors connect to large myelinated A-beta afferent nerve fibres and respond to light mechanical stimulation (Melzack & Wall 1989). In addition, free nerve endings in large numbers are present that respond to all types of stimuli and connect to A-beta, A-delta and C fibres (Melzack & Wall 1984).

Table 2.1 Classification of nerve fibres (adapted and reproduced with kind permission of Appleton and Lange from Ganong W F, Review of Medical Physiology, 17th Edition 1995.)

Fibre type	Number	Diameter (µm)	Conduction velocity (m/s)	Functions
A-alpha	(IA, IB)	12–20	70–120	Proprioception Somatic motor
A-beta	(II)	5–15	40–70	Touch Pressure
A-gamma	(II)	3–6	15–30	Motor to muscle spindles
A-delta	(III)	2–5	12–30	Pain Temperature
B		<3	3–15	Autonomic
C	(IV)	0.5–1.0	0.5–2.3	Sympathetic Pain Pressure Temperature

The large diameter, thickly myelinated A-beta fibres conduct impulses rapidly. The small diameter A-delta fibres have thin myelin sheaths and conduct more slowly. The C fibres, which are merely enveloped by the Schwann cell, are the slowest conducting of all and are called the non-myelinated group. The small A-delta and C fibres are involved in the signalling of painful events.

Stimulation of C fibres produces a dull, diffuse, more deeply perceived burning-type sensation, similar to experimental second (or slow) pain and perhaps the nature of chronic pain, as sufferers often describe their pain in these terms. Selective stimulation of the A-delta fibres produces a sharp prickling sensation, similar to experimental first (or fast) pain and perhaps the nature of acute pain, whereas stimulation of the A-beta fibres produces a sensation of light pressure or tickling (Torebjork & Hallin 1973). However, these results have been challenged by the results of several studies; e.g. Burgess & Perl (1973) found A-delta fibres that were activated by innocuous cutaneous stimuli, and Iggo (1960) found that impulses from the application of non-painful stimuli were also transmitted in unmyelinated C type fibres. Conversely, Willer et al (1978) reported that in man, stimulation of lower limb cutaneous nerves at intensities sufficient to activate only large diameter afferents, resulted in the sensation of prickling pain.

It can therefore be concluded that receptors in the skin are responsive to a variety of stimuli. However, to date, no specific receptor has been associated with a particular type of sensation.

Afferent units

A peripheral nerve fibre and its associated receptors are termed an afferent unit. Echternach (1987) and Wu & Smith (1987) classified afferent units in two ways, into either:

1. high- or low-threshold units, or
2. mechanoreceptive and thermoreceptive.

Those neurons which are activated by both mechanical and thermal stimuli are referred to as polymodal receptive units.

Thermoreceptive units sensitive to both noxious and non-noxious temperatures are common in both animals and humans. Most units respond in a graded manner to increasing or decreasing temperatures and only a few have been found with high-threshold receptors that discharge exclusively at noxious thermal levels (Iggo 1973).

Dubner et al (1975) identified cold- and heat-sensitive units as two distinct populations within the category of thermoreceptive units.

- Transmission of cold stimuli occurs via thermoreceptive units associated with thinly myelinated A-delta fibres.
- Heat thermoreceptive units conduct impulses at both A-delta and C fibre velocities (Iggo 1973).

Like cold thermoreceptors, heat-responsive units discharge in a graded manner, increasing their firing rate with incremental increases in skin temperatures (Dubner et al 1975).

A number of these polymodal nociceptive units are associated with A-delta fibres. These units appear to function in the transmission of 'first' or 'pricking' pain associated with noxious heat stimulation.

Bessou & Perl (1969) identified a group of polymodal nociceptive afferent units which transmit along unmyelinated C fibres. They estimated that approximately 80–90% of C fibre nociceptors are of the polymodal type.

In experiments where only the C fibres were left intact, subjects perceived only the burning or second pain sensation. However, polymodal nociceptors are not activated exclusively by painful stimuli. Van Hees & Gybels (1981) reported sensations following cutaneous activation of C fibre polymodal units.

Sensitization and primary hyperalgesia

C fibre polymodal nociceptors may be involved in pain threshold and tolerance determination. When polymodal nociceptors are stimulated repeatedly or the tissue they innervate is damaged, they show sensitization to further cutaneous stimulation (Wells et al 1988). A-delta nociceptors also sometimes show sensitization but to a lesser degree. Sensitized receptor units are more easily activated by a given stimulus than would otherwise be the case in uninjured skin.

Following the injury there also develops a much larger area of hyperalgesia and allodynia that surrounds the site of injury (secondary hyperalgesia). The mechanisms of sensitization and primary hyperalgesia following injury or inflammation are probably similar and involve endogenous biochemical agents which may play a role in peripheral modulation (Bonica 1990). This is further explained in Chapter 3.

Endogenous biochemical agents travelling along afferent nerve fibres coming from damaged or inflamed tissues may also sensitize wide dynamic range (WDR) central cells (these will be explained later) in the spinal cord so that they respond to almost any peripheral stimulus with a 'pain-type' discharge pattern (Bowsher 1988). That is, they respond abnormally to input from normally innocuous primary afferent messages.

Echternach (1987) suggested that this was due to the sensitization of the WDR cells, either directly or indirectly, by chemical modulator substances released from central terminals within the spinal cord or brain stem in addition to the chemical alteration of primary nociceptive afferents in damaged areas. This may explain why inflamed joints or fractures are very painful even if handled gently, stimulating only low-threshold (nonnociceptive) mechanoreceptors which do not normally give rise to painful sensations.

TRANSMISSION OF NOCICEPTIVE AND NON-NOCICEPTIVE INFORMATION

Mechanism for transmission from receptor cell to nerve fibre

The nociceptive system is normally inactive; however, it becomes active if nociceptive nerve fibres are depolarized by stress, damage, deforming mechanical stimuli or exposure to sufficient quantities of irritating chemical substances (Melzack & Wall 1989, Iggo 1973).

It is thought that the cutaneous free nerve endings contain one or several chemical substances contained within vesicles. These substances are specific and are released in response to a particular stimulation.

Upon appropriate stimulation, the substance is released and diffuses out of the ending to combine with receptor sites on the external surface of the ending, causing depolarization and initiation of the action potential (Bishop 1980). This mechanism of action may be similar to the mechanism involved in synaptic transmission at the postsynaptic membrane: upon release of an adequate amount of receptor substance, interaction is made with the chemically excitable receptor sites. This will cause certain molecular rearrangements and result in opening of the sodium and potassium channels, with an appropriate movement of these ions down their concentration gradients.

There is a greater inward sodium flow than outward potassium flow and so there is a net accumulation of positive charge on the inside of the membrane. If an adequate amount of receptor substance is present, enough sodium will flow in and an excitatory action potential will be initiated (Selkurt 1975).

Many substances have been proposed as possible receptor substances including potassium and ATP released from damaged cells, and histamine, bradykinin and prostaglandins produced in inflamed tissue (Keele & Armstrong 1964). Substance P, an excitatory neurotransmitter has been identified, also lactic acid and 5HT, as have some degrading enzymes whose function it is to remove the receptor substance after its release.

Mechanism of transmission from nerve fibre to spinal cord

If initiated, the nerve action potential or pain impulse is then transmitted to the spinal cord via the nociceptive fibres where they synapse with the neuronal cells in the grey matter in the spinal cord. At spinal levels, afferent cells contribute axons which reach the cord by travelling through segmentally organized dorsal roots (Echternach 1987). Upon reaching the primary afferent terminal, the nerve action potential causes an excitatory neurotransmitter such as substance P to be released (Bishop 1980). Having been released into the synaptic cleft, the neurotransmitter interacts with the chemically excitable receptors on the postsynaptic membrane of the neuronal (or transmitter) cell in the dorsal root and causes electro-physiological alterations in its postsynaptic membrane. If adequate excitatory transmitter substance or receptor substance is released, an action potential will be initiated in the neuronal (transmitter) cell. However, this will depend on the number of occupied receptor sites and hence the number of channels opened, which will in turn depend on the degree of transmitter concentration in the synaptic cleft: the greater the concentration, the greater will be the possibility that the receptors in the synaptic membrane will be occupied. Temporal and spatial summation are also important in the initiation of the postsynaptic action potential (Lamb et al 1980). The transmitter molecule is almost immediately removed from the receptor by a degrading enzyme. The channels then close and the postsynaptic element returns to its resting state.

AFFERENT ORGANIZATION

Neuronal cell bodies concerned with the transmission of impulses to the CNS are located in dorsal root ganglia and selected cranial nerve ganglia.

There are also ventral root afferent fibres. Coggeshall (1979) suggested that up to 27% of the fibres in human ventral roots are unmyelinated and that the majority of these are probably sensory and transmit pain. He also found that of the unmyelinated fibres in the ventral root, half were sensory and half were preganglionic autonomic neurons. Studies of the receptive fields of ventral root afferent fibres indicate that approximately one-third are associated with high-threshold receptors in the body wall (possibly nociceptors). The remaining two-thirds are distributed to visceral structures. Thus visceral and autonomic responses may be associated with pain.

The majority of myelinated and unmyelinated nerve fibres carrying noxious information utilize the dorsal root. As the fibres approach the dorsal root entry zone, a segregation occurs with the large diameter fibres lying dorsomedially and the thin myelinated and unmyelinated fibres lying ventrolaterally (Light & Perl 1979). Within the spinal cord, the majority of these incoming fibres terminate ipsilaterally.

However, axon terminals in the contralateral grey matter have been reported by Culberson et al (1979).

Non-nociceptive information

Figure 2.2 illustrates the transmission of non-nociceptive and nociceptive information to the brain. It should be remembered that non-nociceptive information is transmitted to the spinal cord and brain from the same tissues as nociceptive information.

Large diameter fibres enter the cord medial to Lissauer's tract and bifurcate into ascending and descending branches before they terminate. Thus the large diameter afferents from the lumbosacral regions (including those innervating the corpuscular mechanoreceptors in the skin and in the capsules of the apophyseal and sacroiliac joints and the muscle spindles and tendon organs of the back) enter via the dorsomedial division of the spinal cord (Jayson 1981, Culberson et al 1979).

Most of these large diameter fibres synapse on various spinal cord laminae and about 20% ascend in the fasciculus gracilis and cuneatus where they affect movement and body position (Carpenter et al 1968).

Although most of these fibres are associated with low-threshold sensory units, there are reports of nociceptive responses following their activation, e.g. by Willer (1983).

Nociceptive information

The lateral division of the dorsal root, which contains A-delta and C fibres is thought to play a major role in the transmission of noxious stimuli. The nociceptive afferents from the same tissues of the lumbosacral region are delivered into the spinal cord by way of the ventrolateral division. These

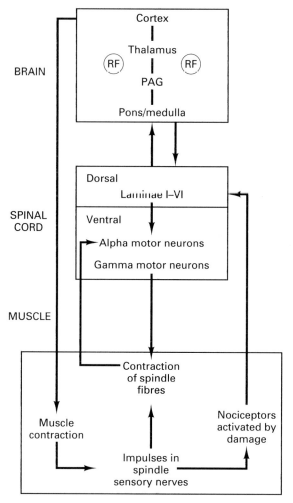

Figure 2.2 Transmission of nociceptive and non-nociceptive information. Key: PAG = periaqueductal grey matter, RF = reticular formation.

afferent fibres enter the spinal cord and occupy the medial portion of Lissauer's tract (Szentagothai 1964).

Upon entering the Lissauer's tract, the axons bifurcate into ascending and descending branches, each of which may travel for one or two segments before terminating in the dorsal horn.

Coggeshall (1979) stated that 80% of the fibres in Lissauer's tract arise from ipsilateral peripheral nerves and the remaining are of propriospinal origin.

Fibres in the medial part of Lissauer's tract have been reported to transmit excitatory impulses, while intrinsic axons occupying the lateral part of

Lissauer's tract appear to convey inhibitory influences from nearby segments. The majority of myelinated and unmyelinated fibres carrying noxious input utilize the dorsal root. As stated previously, there are some ventral root afferent fibres which are involved in nociception and also visceral and autonomic responses associated with pain.

Of the small diameter fibres utilizing the ventrolateral division, some synapse on laminae of the spinal cord, particularly lamina V (Kerr 1975), the axons of which then cross the spinal cord in the anterior grey commissure to turn upwards in the contralateral, anterolateral tracts of the brain to produce the experience of pain. Others project polysynaptically through interneurons in laminae I, VI and VII and ultimately reach the ventrally located motorneuron pools of the back, thigh and abdominal muscles.

Transmission of nociceptive afferent activity through the ascending projection system underlies the evocation of firstly the experience of pain in the lumbosacral region and secondly the simultaneous transmission of activity through the intraspinal polysynaptic system of reflexogenic pathways. This contributes to the changes in motor unit activity in the back, abdominal and lower limb musculature that are associated with nociceptive irritation in the lumbosacral tissues and which result in the clinically apparent disorders of posture and gait (Jayson 1987).

SPINAL ORGANIZATION

Primary afferent neurons involved in the transmission of nociceptive impulses make synaptic contact with neurons in the spinal grey matter and the nucleus caudalis of the spinal trigeminal complex. Cells in different laminae play individual and sometimes unique roles in the processing and transmission of noxious stimuli.

Dorsal

Laminae I–VI, sometimes referred to as the nucleus proprius of the dorsal horn, receive primary afferent fibres from the periphery. Synaptic terminals of peripheral nociceptive afferent fibres are distributed largely to the superficial layers of the dorsal horn. These endings are largely distributed to laminae I–III (Light & Perl 1979).

Lamina I

Lamina I receives noxious input only. A-delta high-threshold mechanical or mechanoreceptors terminate here and also in the lateral part of lamina V. In addition to high-threshold A-delta mechanoreceptors, Perl & Anderson (1978) reported input from A-delta thermoreceptors and polymodal C fibre nociceptors to marginal cells in lamina I. Kerr (1975) suggested that the differential synaptic arrangement in lamina I may be the anatomic substrate for selective excitatory and inhibitory influences.

Lamina II

Lamina II (the substantia gelatinosa) is characterized by an abundance of very small neurons and lack of myelinated fibres marked by densely packed complexes of synaptic endings (Wu & Smith 1987). The axons of substantia gelatinosa (SG) cells have short trajectories with synaptic terminations on the other SG cells at adjacent segments above and below their level of origin. Many of the axons occupy the lateral part of Lissauer's tract and the lateral aspect of the fasciculus proprius. Some SG axons course through the dorsal white commissure to end in lamina II of the contralateral side. Recently, the SG has been divided into an inner and outer zone.

The synaptic terminals in the outer zone have been associated with C fibres from high-threshold thermal nociceptors (Light & Perl 1979), whereas the inner zone is thought to receive information from low-threshold A-delta mechanoreceptors.

Activation of cells in lamina II results in both inhibition and excitation of postsynaptic neurons (Echternach 1987). This would therefore suggest the involvement of neurotransmitter and neuromodulator substances.

Laminae IV, V and VI contain numerous large neurons, many of which give rise to axons contributing to the long ascending spinal pathways.

Lamina IV

The neurons in lamina IV possess dendritic processes which extend into lamina III and the SG. They receive synaptic contacts from low-threshold A-delta fibres (Light & Perl 1979). Cells in lamina IV may be activated by noxious stimuli but **are** more easily and effectively discharged by innocuous tactile stimulation.

Lamina V

Lamina V receives input from noxious and non-noxious primary afferents, i.e. A-beta, A-delta and C fibres (Melzack & Wall 1989). The neurons have large peripheral receptive fields and, because of the above, are known as wide dynamic range (WDR) cells, which were mentioned earlier.

There is also convergence from visceral and somatic receptive units and this may support a theory of referred pain. Convergence of visceral and cutaneous information on to lamina V may constitute part of a mechanism whereby input from one area of the body might influence or modulate the effects of input from another area (Hancock et al 1973). This lamina also contains neurons which respond exclusively to noxious stimulation (Iggo 1973). Afferent fibres terminating in lamina V have been shown to be thinly myelinated A-delta fibres associated with high-threshold mechano-receptors and polymodal nociceptor C fibres (Echternach 1987).

Intermediate

Laminae VII–VIII, sometimes termed the intermediate grey matter, consist of interneurons which neither receive nor project to structures outside the CNS; their input comes from more superficial laminae or from axons descending from higher brain centres.

Although peripheral C fibre input is principally to lamina II, output to the tissue-damage–pain pathway is chiefly from WDR cells in laminae VII and VIII. This means that convergent intraspinal circuitry must exist between input and output and several synapses are known to be involved. This may help to explain why pain elicited by activation of C polymodal nociceptors is less well localized than pinprick sensation, which excites A-delta nociceptors.

Ventral

Lamina IX

The ventral (anterior) horn contains the motor neurons of lamina IX. These axons leave the spinal cord to innervate muscles in the periphery.

Neuropeptides in the spinal cord

There are a number of neuropeptides in the spinal cord which are implicated in the modulation and experience of pain. They are also implicated in somatic and visceral responses to pain. These are further discussed in Chapter 3.

ASCENDING SYSTEMS

The ascending systems transmitting nociceptive information are as follows:

- dorsal column tract (DCT)
- dorsal column postsynaptic system (DCPS)
- multisynaptic ascending system (MAS)
- spinothalamic tract (STT)
- spinoreticular tract (SRT)
- spinomesencephalic tract (SMT)
- trigeminal system (Williams & Warwick 1980).

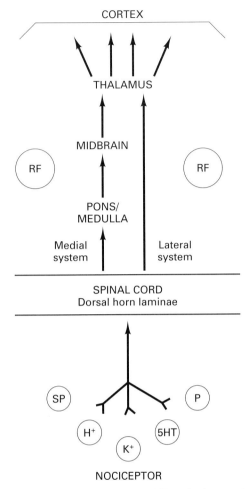

Figure 2.3   Ascending nociceptive pathways. Key: 5HT = 5-hydroxytryptamine (serotonin); H^+ = hydrogen ions; K^+ = potassium ions; P = prostaglandins; SP = substance P.

There are two divisions of the STT, the neospinothalamic tract (nSTT) and the paleospinothalamic tract (pSTT).

The ascending systems can be divided into two major systems known as the lateral and medial system (see Fig. 2.3).

Lateral system

The lateral (lemniscal system) comprises the nSTT, SCT and DCT. The cell bodies of these tracts are found in laminae I and V and project to the posteroventral thalamus and to the somatosensory cortex.

The lateral system is involved with the rapid transmission of phasic discriminative information to quickly bring about a response that prevents further damage.

Medial system

The medial (non-lemniscal) system comprises the pSTT, SRT, STT and MAS. The cell bodies are located in the deeper layer of the spinal grey matter and project to the medial and anterior thalamic nuclei, reticular formation (RF), periaqueductal grey matter (PAG), hypothalamus and limbic forebrain.

The medial system is involved with slower transmission of information. It has been queried by Wyke (1981) as to whether this system is concerned with the determination of arousal and behaviour and whether its activation will prevent further damage and foster rest, protection, care and therefore promote healing and recuperation.

Spinothalamic tract neurons are widely distributed in the dorsal, intermediate and ventral grey regions of the spinal cord. They are involved in the transmission of noxious stimuli. Foreman et al (1979) found that stimulation of A-delta and C fibres or cutaneous stimulation using noxious stimuli activated spinothalamic tract cells. They also found that stimulation in regions of the thalamus activated cervical and lumbar neurons.

A small number of spinothalamic fibres have been identified in the ventral funiculus of the spinal cord, but the role of the ventral spinothalamic tract is unclear (Melzack & Wall 1989).

The spinoreticular tract is also involved in the transmission of noxious stimuli. Le Blanc & Gatipon (1974) found neurons in the brain stem reticular formation to be activated by noxious stimulation. Cells projecting to the brain stem reticular formation have been found in laminae I, IV, V and VI of the dorsal horn as well as in the laminae of the intermediate and ventral grey matter (Ganong 1989). As the spinoreticular tract has similar laminar origins to the spinothalamic, Perl & Anderson (1980) suggested that its fibres represent collateral branches of spinothalamic tract axons. However, spinal neurons have been found with projections limited to nuclei of the brain stem reticular formation (Perl & Anderson 1980). The reticular formation of the brain stem appears to represent a relay point for noxious impulses. It projects on to the intralaminar nucleus of the thalamus and also to the hypothalamus (Bowsher 1988). The diffuse projections of the medial system and also the involvement of neuropeptides, including serotonin and substance P, at various sites implies a role in biochemically-mediated behavioural, autonomic and possibly endocrinological responses to pain.

BRAIN STEM

Pons and medulla

These structures have been implicated in the processing of nociceptive information in addition to their roles of maintaining functions such as breathing and heart rate. Mediation may be via reticular neurons and this may be why breathing and heart rate are affected in conditions of severe pain.

MIDBRAIN

Periaqueductal grey (PAG) and periventricular grey (PVG) matter

These areas of the midbrain are rich in opioid and non-opioid peptides which play an important role in the modulation of pain. In addition, this region is an important component of the descending pain control system which is covered in Chapter 3.

BASAL GANGLIA

The involvement of the basal ganglia in motor functions is well known. However, recent neurophysiological, clinical and behavioural studies have indicated that the basal ganglia also process non-nociceptive and nociceptive somatosensory information (Chudler & Dong 1995). Some neurons within the basal ganglia encode stimulus intensity but are not involved with encoding the location of the stimulus.

Neuroanatomical studies have also indicated that the basal ganglia are rich in many different neuroactive chemicals, such as met-enkephalin, substance P, dopamine and GABA, that may be involved in the modulation of nociceptive information. (Modulation of pain will be presented in a later chapter.) The reduction of pain behaviour following electrical stimulation of the substantia nigra and caudate nucleus provides additional evidence for a role of the basal ganglia in pain modulation. Some patients with basal ganglia disease such as Parkinson's disease have alterations in pain sensation in addition to motor abnormalities. Frequently these patients have intermittent pain that is difficult to localize.

Chudler & Dong (1995) suggest that the basal ganglia may be involved in the following:

* sensory–discriminative dimension of pain
* affective dimension of pain
* cognitive dimension of pain
* modulation of nociceptive information
* sensory gating of nociceptive information to higher motor areas.

THALAMIC NOCICEPTIVE DISPERSAL SYSTEM

Ascending pathways from the spinal cord and brain stem which transmit nociceptive information terminate in the thalamus after coursing through the brain stem, reticular formation and midbrain. The synaptic endings of these pathways are distributed to the posteroventral, medial and anterior thalamic nuclei, pulvinar and secondary thalamic nuclei (Jayson 1987).

Posteroventral thalamus

The main sources of afferent input are from the dorsal column (gracile and cuneate) nuclei, cervicothalamic tracts and spinothalamic tracts (Bowsher 1988). It responds mainly to the application of innocuous tactile and thermal stimuli, and only a few units are responsive to noxious stimuli. Electrical stimulation of the posteroventral thalamus produces localized pain (Halliday & Logue 1972). Therefore nociceptive information entering the ventrobasal nuclei of the thalamus is important in the sensory discriminative aspects of pain, i.e. the location of a particular stimulus.

These areas project axons to the primary and secondary somatosensory cortices (Melzack & Wall 1989).

This region of the thalamus contains more neurons responsive to noxious stimuli and has bilateral receptive fields.

Ascending projections in the anterolateral tracts which terminate in the posteroventral thalamus are referred to as the neospinothalamic system (Echternach 1987). Activation of this system provides information about the location of the stimulus and its physical character (e.g. sharp, hot, intense, brief).

The medial and anterior thalamic nuclei

These receive direct spinal projections (Stein 1982). Ascending projections which terminate in this region are referred to as the paleospinothalamic system (Melzack & Wall 1989). Cells giving rise to spinothalamic axons terminating on these nuclei originate in laminae I and V, intermediate and ventral horns. The input to this region comes from the spinothalamic tract and there is also synaptic input from nuclei of the brain stem reticular formation. It can therefore be activated by a direct pathway (spinothalamic) and by a multisynaptic route (spinoreticulothalamic). From this area, axons are projected to the frontal cortex, cingulate cortex and the limbic system. Activation of this system brings about the feeling of 'hurt' and the emotional experience of the painful stimulus.

Medial thalamic nuclei and pulvinar

These nuclei contain neurons which project axons to the temporal lobe. Activation of this system brings about the memory of past painful experiences.

Secondary and medial thalamic nuclei

This region contains neurons which projects axons to hypothalamic nuclei. Activation of this system brings about visceral hormonal effects associated with acute and chronic pain.

RETICULAR INVOLVEMENT

The reticular formation receives convergent information channels from all the principal parts of the nervous system and, in turn, it projects directly or indirectly back to all these regions, modulating their activities through complex and ill-understood mechanisms that involve synaptic neuro-transmission and local neuroparacrine as well as neuroendocrine effects.

Much of the reticular formation is non-specific and for this reason it influences many diverse functions and behaviours including an effect on pain perception and response.

Functional associations of the reticular formation

The RF is often associated with sleep, arousal, states of consciousness and perception. The descending serotonergic bulbospinal fibres from the nucleus raphe and noradrenergic fibres from the locus coeruleus in the pons are held responsible for the relaxation of limb and trunk musculature during REM sleep.

In addition, the RF is associated with:

- somatomotor control
- somatosensory control
- visceromotor control.

Somatomotor control

This is achieved through the reticulospinal tracts originating from the medial two-thirds of the pontomedullary reticular formation.

The serotonergic bulbospinal fibres from the raphe have been held as mediating the general relaxation of body musculature that characterizes REM sleep.

Groups of the foregoing reticular neurons controlling the motor neuron pools innervating the diaphragm and intercostal musculature have been said to constitute the hierarchy of respiratory 'centres' (Williams & Warwick 1980).

There are additionally many indirect influences of the RF on somatomotor control. These include reticular inputs to the cerebellum and other brain stem complexes including the olivary nuclei, colliculi, red nucleus, substantia nigra, corpus striatum, thalamus, subthalamic nuclei and somatomotor cortex.

Somatosensory control

The RF exerts influence over pain perception through its projections to thalamic, cortical and sub-cortical structures and it also provides input to the special senses. The extensive RF nuclei act as an integrative area where ascending normal sensory and nociceptive relays interact with cortical, limbic and thalamic input. These interactions may partly explain the emotional and visceral hormonal reactions to pain and thus the variability of the subjective report of pain experience. Cognitive and emotional factors may be used to reduce the intensity of pain from whatever cause via the reticular formation nuclei, and this may partly explain analgesia as a result of psychological methods of pain control (Elton et al 1983).

It appears that nuclear areas of the brain stem RF can influence pain perception by decreasing the activity in the ascending nociceptive pathways. Since many of the ascending pathways terminate in or send collateral branches to the brain stem RF, a negative feedback system can be established whereby nociceptive impulses transmitted in the antero-lateral tracts stimulate brain stem nuclei which in turn decrease activity in the originally stimulated anterolateral tract neurons (Gebhart et al 1983).

Visceromotor control

Preganglionic neuronal somata and dendrites of non-striated muscle are controlled either directly or indirectly by reticulobulbar and descending reticulospinal fibres. This includes input to the cardiovascular system and to the thoraco-abdominal viscera.

Forebrain control of autonomic activities involves areas of the frontal and cingulate cortices, the major limbic structures (olfactory nerves, bulb and tract, amygdaloid complex, septal areas and hippocampus), dorsal thalamic nuclei, hypothalamic nuclei and descending fascicles of the various tegmental bundles with destinations in the RF (via the reticulo-bulbar and reticulospinal tracts).

Other functions of the RF include neuroendocrine transduction through input to the hypothalamus and pineal gland, the maintenance of circadian rhythms and learning and memory.

All hypothalamic nuclei and limbic structures receive widespread input from both aminergic and non-aminergic elements of the RF. Surgical or pharmacological manipulation of these brain stem reticular elements causes profound alterations in these diverse aspects of complex behaviour.

The reticular formation in the brain stem discharges impulses continually and exerts an inhibitory effect on pain by closing the gate in the substantia gelatinosa via the reticulospinal tract. Increasing reticular inhibitory activity will thus decrease the experience of pain. This is discussed in a later chapter.

CORTICAL INVOLVEMENT

The cortex also plays a role in the processing of pain and has a role in sensory–discriminative and the emotional/affective dimensions of pain (Kenshalo & Willis 1991).

A small number of cells have been found in the somatosensory cortex that respond to noxious stimulation (Lamour et al 1982).

Thalamic projections from the ventrobasal complex, part of the medial group of thalamic nuclei and possibly the posterior group, to specific nociceptive neurons in the somatosensory cortex may be important in sensory discriminative components of pain. The somatosensory areas I and II and the frontal and limbic lobes, which are involved in somatic motor function and control of emotional behaviour, are influenced by thalamic nociceptive neurons. It is possible that nociceptive input to these areas may be important in producing affective responses to a particular stimulus and the inhibition, if appropriate, of avoidance and escape behaviour. The existence of significant medial thalamic projections to the hypothalamus could account for the autonomic reactions commonly seen in association with acute and chronic pain syndromes. It is possible that the medial and intralaminar nuclei, together with many subcortical and cortical areas (other than somatosensory areas I and II), play an important role in the motivational–affective reactions to painful stimuli (Echternach 1987, Wu & Smith 1987). The cingulate cortex has also been implicated in the affective dimensions of pain (Chudler & Dong 1995). Recent studies using positron emission tomography in humans have demonstrated that painful thermal stimulation produces a significant increase in blood flow to the anterior cingulate cortex. In animals, electrical stimulation has been found to evoke vocalization which also suggests its involvement in affective behaviours (Talbot et al 1991).

The cortex regulates the activity of the reticular formation by way of corticoreticular fibres and exerts both a facilitatory and inhibitory influence.

Variation in the activity of this system may underlie the changes in awareness of peripheral nociceptive stimuli that are associated with alteration in the direction of attention and the induction of hypnosis. Cortical activity is augmented by anxiety and reduced by emotional tranquillity. This is further discussed in a later chapter.

DESCENDING SYSTEMS

The descending pathways involved in nociception are:

- corticospinal
- reticulospinal
- multiple bulbospinal systems.

Corticospinal

The corticospinal tract originating from the sensory cortex synapses on laminae I–VII, whereas that originating from the motor cortex synapses on laminae VI–IX.

The corticospinal tract is usually associated with patterns of voluntary movement; however, some 40% of its fibres are sensory afferents from the cerebral cortex and may exert an inhibitory action by willed distraction away from the pain (Charman 1989).

Reticulospinal

The reticulospinal tract originates in the nucleus gigantocellularis and synapses on laminae I, II and V–VIII. Presynaptic inhibitory effects, which probably involve 5HT as a transmitting agent, are exerted on the nociceptive afferent terminals subtended on the projection neurons in lamina V. Interneurons of the RF projections exert a facilitatory influence on these neutrons. Since many of these ascending pathways terminate in or send collateral branches to the brain stem RF, a negative feedback system can be established whereby nociceptive impulses transmitted in the anterolateral tracts stimulate brain stem nuclei which then reduce activity in the originally stimulated anterolateral neurons. Reticular activity can thus be selectively augmented or reduced.

Multiple bulbospinal systems

There are many transmitters and pathways involved in bulbospinal systems (Dubner & Bennett 1983, Le Blanc & Gatipon 1974). Not only are there multiple brain stem sources of axons in the dorsolateral funiculus, but within the rostroventral medulla (RVM) there are cells with different transmitters. Thus there are neurons in the RVM that contain 5HT, substance P, enkephalin, thyrotropin-releasing hormone or almost any combination of the four (Basbaum 1985). Furthermore, 5HT, substance P and enkephalin are present in RVM cells that project to the spinal cord. In addition to providing separate pathways to the spinal cord, these parallel systems also interact at the brain stem and spinal levels.

Descending pain control system

This endogenous system is mediated by opiate and catecholaminergic fibres. It projects from cortical areas to the PAG and PVG of the midbrain, to the brain stem and to the spinal and medullary dorsal horn (Bonica 1990).

Chapter 3 reviews the biochemistry of pain and details this system.

THE AUTONOMIC NERVOUS SYSTEM AND PAIN

The autonomic nervous system (ANS) is also implicated in the experience of pain as sympathetic nerve fibres synapse in the dorsal root of the spinal cord along with somatic neurons from peripheral nerves. Information in these pathways may be carried to the periphery where there may be sympathetic autonomic effects such as vasoconstriction, or may travel onwards in the multisynaptic ascending system (MAS) to the reticular formation, hypothalamus and limbic system. Thus there may be diverse autonomic effects in response to the experience of pain, such as a feeling of nausea, sweating and feeling dizzy. It has been suggested that abnormal neural circuitry in these pathways may be responsible for neuralgic pain (Bond 1984).

Summary

Nociceptive and non-nociceptive information from the lumbosacral region is transmitted from the periphery to the spinal cord. This nociceptive information is transmitted onwards to higher centres of the brain which produce the experience and response to pain and also produce changes in motor unit activity which results in clinically apparent disorders of posture and gait.

SUMMARY OF MAIN POINTS

1. The lumbosacral nociceptor receptor systems are found in skin, subcutaneous and adipose tissue, capsule of the facet and sacroiliac joints, ligaments, dura mater and the walls of the intramuscular arteries within the lumbosacral muscles. The nociceptive system becomes active if nociceptive nerve fibres are depolarized by stress, damage, deforming mechanical stimuli or exposure to sufficient quantities of irritating chemical substances.

2. Polymodal C fibre nociceptors are found in the deeper parts of the skin and virtually every other tissue. They are frequently sensitive to mechanical, thermal and chemical noxious stimuli. 80–90% of C fibre nociceptors are of the polymodal type.

3. Receptors in the skin are responsive to a variety of stimuli. However, to date, no specific receptor has been associated with a particular type of sensation.

4. A peripheral nerve fibre and its associated receptors are termed an afferent unit. Afferent units are classified into either high- or low-threshold units or mechanoreceptive and thermoreceptive.

5. Stimulation of A-beta fibres produces a sensation of light pressure or tickling. Stimulation of A-delta fibres produces a sharp, prickling sensation similar to acute pain and experimental first pain. Stimulation of C fibres

produces a dull diffuse more deeply perceived burning-type sensation, similar to chronic pain and experimental second (or slow) pain.

6. When a cell is damaged there is a release of potassium ions and a synthesis of prostaglandins and bradykinin. Impulses generated in the stimulated terminal propagate not only to the spinal cord but into other terminal branches where they induce the release of peptides including substance P. With continued liberation of substance P, the levels of histamine continue to rise in the extracellular fluid (ECF) and indirectly sensitize nearby nociceptors. Sensitization leads to a gradual spread of hyperalgesia and/or tenderness.

7. The majority of myelinated and unmyelinated nerve fibres carrying noxious information utilize the dorsal root. As the fibres approach the dorsal root entry zone, a segregation occurs so that the large diameter, non-nociceptive fibres lie dorsomedially and the thinly myelinated and unmyelinated, nociceptive fibres lie ventrolaterally.

8. Of the small diameter unmyelinated fibres utilizing the ventrolateral division, some synapse on laminae of the spinal cord. The axons then cross the spinal cord and ascend in the anterolateral tracts of the brain to produce the experience of pain. Others project polysynaptically through interneurons in laminae I, VI and VII and ultimately reach the ventrally located motorneuron pools of the back, thigh and abdominal muscles.

9. Transmission of nociceptive afferent activity through the ascending projection system underlies the evocation of firstly the experience of pain in the lumbosacral region and secondly the simultaneous transmission of activity through the intraspinal polysynaptic system of reflexogenic pathways. This contributes to the changes in the back, abdominal and lower limb musculature that are associated with nociceptive irritation in the lumbosacral tissues and which result in the clinically apparent disorders of posture and gait.

10. Cells in different laminae of the spinal cord play individual and sometimes unique roles in the processing and transmission of noxious stimuli. Laminae I–VI receive nociceptive and non-nociceptive primary afferent fibres from the periphery, laminae VII–VIII receive input from more superficial laminae or from axons descending from higher brain centres, and axons from laminae IX–X leave the spinal cord to innervate muscles in the periphery.

11. The ascending nociceptive systems can be divided into two major systems known as the medial and lateral system.

The lateral (lemniscal) system comprises the nSTT, SCT and DCT. The cell bodies of these tracts are found in laminae I and V and project to the posteroventral thalamus and to the somatosensory cortex. The lateral system is involved with the rapid transmission of phasic discriminative information to quickly bring about a response to prevent further damage.

The medial (non-lemniscal) system comprises the pSTT, SRT and MAS. The cell bodies are located in the deeper layer of the spinal grey matter and project to the medial and anterior thalamic nuclei, reticular formation, PAG, hypothalamus and limbic forebrain. The medial system is involved with the slower transmission of information. It is suggested that this system is concerned with the determination of arousal and behaviour and will influence behaviour to rest and recuperate and thus facilitate healing.

12. Ascending pathways from the spinal cord and brain stem which transmit nociceptive information terminate in the thalamus after coursing through the brain stem, RF and midbrain. The synaptic endings of these pathways are distributed to the posteroventral, medial and anterior thalamic nuclei, pulvinar and secondary thalamic nuclei.

Projections from the posteroventral thalamus project to areas of the cerebral cortex and are concerned with the location and qualitative nature of the painful stimulus, whereas projections from the medial and anterior thalamic nuclei project to the frontal cortex, cingulate cortex and limbic system and are concerned with the feeling of 'hurt' and the emotional experience of the painful stimulus.

Projections from the medial thalamic nuclei and pulvinar project to the temporal lobe and are concerned with the memory of past painful experience.

Projections from the secondary and medial thalamic nuclei project to hypothalamic nuclei and bring about the visceral–hormonal effects associated with acute and chronic pain.

13. Neural tracts from many sensory systems synapse with each other in the RF nuclei. Much of the RF is non-specific and for this reason it influences many diverse functions and behaviours. The RF exerts an influence over pain perception through its projections to thalamic, cortical and subcortical structures and exerts an effect on somatomotor control through the reticulospinal tracts originating from the pontomedullary RF. In addition, the serotonergic bulbospinal fibres from the raphe have been held as mediating the general relaxation of body musculature that characterizes REM sleep. There are additionally many indirect influences of the RF on somatomotor control.

The extensive RF nuclei act as an integrative area where ascending normal sensory and nociceptive relays interact with cortical, limbic and thalamic input. These interactions may partly explain the emotional and visceral hormonal reaction to pain and thus the variability of the subjective report of the pain experience. Cognitive and emotional factors may be used to reduce the intensity of pain via the RF and this may explain analgesia as a result of psychological methods of pain control.

Nuclear areas of the brain stem RF may influence pain perception by decreasing the activity in the ascending nociceptive pathways through a negative feedback circuit.

14. The cortex regulates the activity of the RF by way of corticoreticular fibres and exerts both a facilitatory and inhibitory influence.

15. The descending pathways involved in nociception are the cortico-spinal tract, reticulospinal tract and multiple bulbospinal systems. There is also a descending pain control system which projects from cortical areas to the PAG and PVG of the midbrain, to the brain stem and to the spinal and medullary dorsal horn. This system is mediated by opiate and catecholaminergic fibres.

Biochemical factors in pain

Nicola Adams

INTRODUCTION

The previous sections have been concerned with neurophysiological mechanisms involved in pain production. This chapter aims to review biochemical aspects of pain as various neurotransmitters and peptides are involved in the production of the experience of pain. These neurotransmitters exert effects on perception and response to pain and biochemical factors are then, in turn, affected by these psychological factors.

In order to appreciate these interactions, it is first necessary to understand the way in which biochemical factors are involved in pain production.

ENDOGENOUS BIOCHEMICAL AGENTS (MEDIATORS)

Tissue damage caused by injury, disease or inflammation releases endogenous chemicals called algogenic, algesic or pain-producing substances, such as hydrogen ions, potassium ions, serotonin, histamine, prostaglandins, bradykinin and substance P, into the extracellular fluid that surrounds the nociceptors (Bonica 1990).

Keele & Armstrong (1964) concluded from 'blister base' experiments that these substances play a causal role in pain associated with inflammation, trauma, bone tumours, ischaemia and a variety of other pathophysiological conditions. In addition to direct excitatory action on the membrane of nociceptors, these agents may have an indirect excitatory action by altering the local microcirculation. Depending on the algesic substance, there may be either vasoconstriction or vasodilation and increased capillary permeability. Increased capillary permeability permits extravasation of additional neuroactive or vasoactive substances such as the plasma kinins and serotonin. These in turn disturb the physiological and chemical microenvironment of nociceptors and thus further increase nociceptive excitability. Continued release of these chemical mediators may cause continued stimulation and sensitization (hyperalgesia) until complete healing of the injured tissue (Melzack & Wall 1989).

What happens when a cell is damaged?

When a cell is damaged there is release of potassium ions and a synthesis of prostaglandins and bradykinin (Fig. 3.1A). Prostaglandins increase the sensitivity of the terminal to bradykinin and other pain-producing substances. Impulses generated in the stimulated terminal propagate not only to the spinal cord but also into terminal branches where they induce the release of peptides, including substance P (Fig. 3.1B). This peptide causes vasodilation and neurogenic oedema with further accumulation of bradykinin, and also causes release of histamine from mast cells and serotonin (5HT) from platelets. With continued liberation of substance P, the levels of histamine and serotonin continue to rise in the extracellular fluid and indirectly sensitize nearby nociceptors (Fig. 3.1C). Sensitization leads to a gradual spread of hyperalgesia and/or tenderness (Bonica 1990).

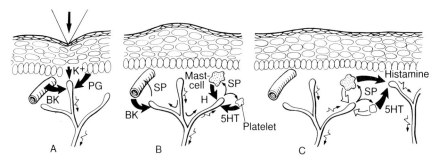

Figure 3.1   Sequence of events in cellular damage. Key: 5HT = 5-hydroxytryptamine (serotonin); BK = bradykinin; H = histamine; K^+ = potassium ions; PG = prostaglandins; SP = substance P.

Source of endogenous chemicals

Serotonin, histamine, potassium, hydrogen ions, prostaglandins and other members of the arachidonic cascade are found in the tissues (Ganong 1989). Kinins are found in plasma and substance P is found at nerve terminals (Maule et al 1989). Histamine is found in the granules of mast cells, in basophils and platelets and serotonin is present in mast cells and platelets (Yaksh & Hammond 1982).

Release of these amines may be induced by mechanical injury, noxious heat, radiation and certain byproducts of tissue damage such as thrombin, collagen and adrenaline. Tissue damage also induces release of lipidic acids of the arachidonic acid cascade, such as the leukotrienes, the prostaglandins and the slow-reacting substance of anaphylaxis (SRSA) (Yaksh & Hammond 1982, Morrison & Henson 1978).

Bradykinin produces increased vascular permeability, promotes vasodilation, induces leucocyte chemotaxis and activates nociceptors. The action of bradykinin on nociceptors is brought about by prostaglandins present in the injured tissue compartments. In damaged skin, there is a marked elevation of prostanoid levels, which is blocked by cyclo-oxygenase (Winkelman 1968). Thus non-steroidal anti-inflammatory drugs (NSAIDs) are effective in the treatment of acute pain due to tissue trauma.

Neurotransmitters in primary afferents and the spinal cord

It is likely that there are many types of neurotransmitters in the central terminals of primary afferents (Yaksh 1986, Hokfelt 1983). The most important are glutamate and aspartate, found in large dorsal root ganglion (DRG) cells and a number of agents found in small cells of the DRG including fluoride-resistant acid phosphatase (FRAP) and a number of peptides such as substance P, vasoactive intestinal peptide (VIP), somatostatin, cholecystokinin (CCK), gastrin-releasing peptide, angiotensin II, calcitonin gene related peptide (CGRP), leu-enkephalin (ENK) and dynorphin (DYN) (Devlin 1986). These are shown in Table 3.1.

Thus a number of neurotransmitters are involved in the production of pain and the so-called 'gut peptides' are implicated in the modulation and experience of pain. This may also explain some of the somatic and visceral responses to pain.

Both opioid and non-opioid peptides are involved in the modulation of pain at various locations in the neuraxis.

ENDOGENOUS OPIOID PEPTIDES

This group includes methionine, leu-enkephalin, beta-endorphin and dynorphin. They have been studied in relation to their role in the

Table 3.1 Neuropeptides present within the central nervous system

Neuropeptide	Location
Substance P	Laminae I–III, V PAG, limbic system, brain stem Thalamus, hypothalamus, amygdaloid
Cholecystokinin (CCK)	Laminae I–III Neocortex, limbic system, amygdaloid
Vasoactive intestinal polypeptide (VIP)	Laminae I, V Neocortex, amygdaloid
Somatostatin	Laminae I–III Neocortex, hypothalamus, amygdaloid Limbic system, brain stem
Dynorphin Enkephalin	Laminae I–III, V PAG, hypothalamus, brain stem

perception of pain and also have been used in the treatment of pain. Endorphins have also been implicated in the mediation of placebo analgesia

There are several types of distinct opiate receptor, mu (morphine), delta (enkephalins), kappa (dynorphin) and epsilon (beta-endorphin), and a common high-affinity receptor with mainly analgesic properties. Each type has its own analgesic potencies, withdrawal syndromes and binding characteristics. They play a role in a number of physiological processes including pain perception, pain tolerance, thermoregulation, eating, learning, sexual behaviour and the regulation of central cardiovascular control and respiration (Elton et al 1983).

Beta-endorphin, given intraventricularly in rats, results in analgesia lasting 30–60 minutes. Larger doses may result in rigid immobility, loss of reflexes, changes in body temperature and other behavioural changes.

As opioids are inhibited by naloxone, an opiate antagonist, naloxone has been used in many studies to determine the presence of opioid peptides.

Hughes (1975) identified endorphins and enkephalins in several areas of the brain, particularly the PAG and PVG of the midbrain. These areas are the most effective in stimulation-produced analgesia (SPA). In addition, there has been evidence that local opioid systems exist at the level of the spinal cord and this led to the development of intraspinal narcotic analgesia therapy (Yaksh & Rudy 1978).

It has been shown that opioids inhibit release of substance P and have an inhibitory effect on pain.

The opioids play an important role in the descending pain control system which is reviewed later (p. 42).

CSF endorphin levels are lower in patients with chronic pain and with low pain thresholds. Levels of endorphins also increase in the CSF after acupuncture and analgesic CNS stimulation (Recht & Abrams 1986). A congenital overabundance of opioid peptides has been hypothesized as mediating the inability to feel pain (Capper 1986).

Research into enkephalin-like opioid production in the adrenal medulla has suggested relationships between psychophysiological reactions and clinical states. There is a complex set of relationships between opioids, catecholamines, stress, mood and pain. These mechanisms may be disturbed in certain subjects with resultant physiological and psychological symptoms.

NON-OPIOID PEPTIDES

This group includes substance P (SP), neurokinin A, neurokinin B, cholecystokinin (CCK), vasoactive intestinal polypeptide (VIP) and somatostatin. Some are present in dorsal horn intrinsic neurons, notably the substantia gelatinosa, in lamina II. Thus they are involved in modulation at this level.

Cells excited by substance P are often activated naturally by noxious radiant heat, strong mechanical stimuli and intra-arterial injection of bradykinin (Cuello & Matthews 1989). Frequently SP facilitates the response of cells activated by noxious cutaneous stimuli. There is an inverse correlation between activity in afferents that contain substance P, somatostatin, VIP, CCK and/or FRAP and the animal's response to otherwise aversive chemical and thermal stimuli.

Substance P

This neuropeptide is found in unmyelinated primary neurons and their terminals (Cuello & Matthews 1989) and in many regions of the central and peripheral nervous system (Maule et al 1989).

Substance P has been demonstrated in the peripheral terminals of unmyelinated primary afferents which supply human skin, sweat glands, glands of the nasal mucosa, small blood vessels in the skin and the pulmonary circuit, coronary and cerebral vessels, tooth pulp and the eye (Cuello & Matthews 1989). In addition, Parris et al (1990) demonstrated the presence of substance P in saliva.

It has been postulated that the primary event in migraine is a spontaneous discharge in the trigeminal nerve pathways with release of substance P from trigeminal nerve branches which may add a vascular component to migraine headache (Yaksh & Aimone 1990). Visceral and autonomic terminals possess stores of substance P that are associated with primary afferents. Substance P immunoreactive sensory fibres also supply the gastrointestinal (GI) tract, the ureters and the trigone neck of the urinary bladder. These substance P sensory fibres may be responsible for conveying nociceptive information from the viscera and perhaps also act locally in inducing vasodilation (Cuello & Matthews 1989). Substance P may also be involved in somatovisceral reflexes and referred pain.

Parris et al (1990) found that both saliva and plasma levels of immuno-reactive SP were lower in patients with chronic low back pain than in healthy volunteers. Cerebrospinal fluid (CSF) levels of SP in patients with chronic pain have been shown by Almay et al (1988) to be lower than CSF levels of SP in healthy human volunteers. Rimon et al (1984) found an elevation of SP-like immunoreactivity in the CSF of psychiatric patients, though it was not specified whether these patients also complained of chronic pain.

Substance P therefore plays an integral role in the pain process. Its distribution in the unmyelinated fibres, spinal cord laminae, PAG and nucleus raphe dorsalis (NRD) and visceral and autonomic terminals implies the role of this peptide with regard to the initiation and pro-pagation of the pain impulse and also in the neural circuitry that sustains chronic pain. Through its interactions with opioids and other peptides, it would appear to facilitate nociceptive impulses with their associated visceral and autonomic effects, and may be involved in the phenomenon of referred pain. In addition, Yaksh & Aimone (1990) and Ganong (1989) suggested that substance P may exert an effect on catecholamines such as serotonin which has been found by Ward & Bloom (1982) to be implicated in depression. Thus SP may indirectly affect the psychological reactivity to chronic pain. Its facilitatory effect on nociception appears to be through the enhancement of a conventional yet unknown neurotransmitter.

Other peptides

Somatostatin derives from a population of small diameter dorsal root ganglion cells and from somatostatin cell bodies within lamina II, and exerts a predominantly inhibitory effect on nociceptors (Ganong 1989).

Neurotensin may activate other intrinsic neurons of the dorsal horn that, in turn, presynaptically control the release of substance P from primary afferent fibres.

NEUROCHEMISTRY AND EMOTION—THE ROLE OF MONOAMINES

The mechanisms involved in the relationship of opioid and non-opioid peptides to behavioural and emotional responses is unclear. Opioids are known to induce a feeling of euphoria in addition to their analgesic pro-perties. It is thought that they may exert an effect on monoamine trans-mitters, which have been implicated in mood.

The monoamine transmitters in the brain are related to emotional responses and their distribution has been mapped using histochemical techniques (Ganong 1989, Devlin 1986).

Monoamines that have been implicated in mood include:

- serotonin
- noradrenaline
- acetylcholine
- gamma-aminobutyric acid (GABA).

Serotonin

Serotonin has been implicated in both chronic pain and depression, and sleep disturbance which is characteristic of depression. Many patients with chronic pain also complain of sleep disturbance. Antidepressant drugs which increase the amount of serotonin available at brain synapses have been successful in the treatment of depression and also of chronic pain (Blumer & Heilbronn 1982).

Serotonergic neurons discharge rapidly in the awake state, slowly during drowsiness, more slowly with bursts during sleep and not at all during REM sleep. The activity of serotonergic neurons is depressed by lysergic acid diethylamide (LSD) and it has been postulated by Ganong (1989) that the psychotomimetic response to LSD is in effect dreaming in the awake state. However, the relation of serotonin to mental functions remains uncertain. Descending serotonergic fibre systems may inhibit transmission in pain pathways of the dorsal horn (Messing & Lyttle 1977).

The relationship between chronic pain and depression is unclear and this may be because this neurotransmitter is implicated in both conditions.

Noradrenaline

The distribution of noradrenaline in the brain parallels that of serotonin (Ganong 1989, Guyton 1986). Studies with drugs that affect noradrenaline indicate that mood is related to the amount of free noradrenaline available at synapses in the brain. When too little noradrenaline is available, depression may result (Baldessarini 1975). Drugs such as monoamine oxidase inhibitors and amphetamine elevate mood by increasing free noradrenaline (Rogers et al 1985). The tricyclic antidepressants decrease the reuptake of liberated noradrenaline, thus leaving more available to act on the postsynaptic structures (Walsh 1983).

Descending serotonin and noradrenaline-containing axons which arise from a relatively small number of neurons in the brain stem are distributed to widespread regions of the medullary and spinal dorsal horn and give off a number of boutons along their paths through the spinal cord.

Dubner & Bennett (1983) suggested that the multitargeted effects of these neurons provide a global enhancement or suppression that enables dorsal horns to respond more effectively to incoming sensory information. They believed that such mechanisms probably form the neural basis of attentional mechanisms and the ability of animals and humans to extract behaviourally relevant information from the environment.

Acetylcholine

Acetylcholine is distributed throughout the CNS, with high concentrations in the cerebral cortex, thalamus and various nuclei in the basal forebrain. There are some projections to the olfactory bulb, amygdala and neocortex and these projections may be involved in motivation, perception and cognition (Strongman 1987). Other cholinergic neurons, through their projections, may be involved in the attention and arousal functions of the ascending reticular system (Guyton 1986).

GABA

Recent research has shown that the peptide, gamma-aminobutyric acid (GABA), has been implicated in anxiety states (Devlin 1986). Although research has been mainly carried out using animal models, findings have been generalized to a human population.

Thus it can be seen that disturbance of neurotransmitters can cause profound alterations in mood. In turn, mood alterations may cause greater or lesser amounts of these neurotransmitters to be produced. As these neurotransmitters are also involved in other functions such as cognitive activity and pain perception, any disturbance will cause an effect on these processes and vice versa.

Thus psychological processes are interrelated with neurochemical processes and therefore a clearer relationship emerges of the way in which a person in pain may become depressed or the way in which a depressed person may develop pain.

CIRCUITRY AND NEUROCHEMISTRY OF THE DESCENDING PAIN CONTROL SYSTEM

As mentioned earlier, an endogenous pain control system exists which can inhibit pain. A number of opioid and non-opioid peptides and mono-amine transmitters are involved in this system.

The models of the descending inhibitory system that have evolved consist of four, tiered CNS parts (Fig. 3.2) (Bonica 1990).

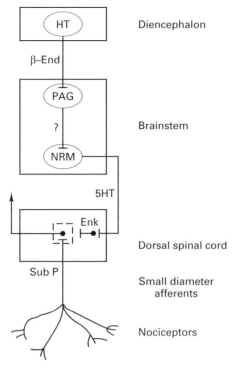

Figure 3.2   Descending pain control system (after Bowsher 1988). Key: 5HT =
5-hydroxytryptamine (serotonin); β-End = beta-endorphin; Enk = enkephalin;
HT = hypothalamus; NRM = nucleus raphe magnus; PAG = periaqueductal grey matter;
Sub P = substance P.

1. Cortical and diencephalic systems.

2. Mesencephalic PAG and PVG which are rich in enkephalins and opiate receptors and can be activated by electrical stimulation or micro-injection of small amounts of opiates.

3. Parts of the rostroventral medulla especially the nucleus raphe magnus (NRM) and adjacent nuclei which receive excitatory input from the PAG and in turn send serotonergic and noradrenergic fibres via the dorsolateral funiculus, that project to the spinal and medullary dorsal horn.

4. The spinal and medullary dorsal horn, which receives terminals of axons from the NRM and adjacent nuclei. These descending fibres are serotonergic and terminate among nociceptive transmission cells in laminae I, II and V and thus selectively inhibit nociceptor neurons, includ-ing interneurons and the ascending STT, SRT and SMT.

There is also evidence that noradrenaline-containing neurons originating in the locus coeruleus and other brain stem sites contribute to this endo-genous pain system.

Cortical and diencephalic systems

The descending systems are the corticoreticular tract, corticospinal tract, raphespinal and bulbospinal tracts.

Cognitive and motivational processes involve activity of complex and variable parts of the cerebrum and play an important role in stress-induced analgesia, such as when an athlete continues running in a race when he or she has a sprained ankle. Although the pathways and neuro-transmitters are not known, it is likely that they enhance the inhibitory function of the mesencephalic and medullary structures.

Diencephalic structures involved in transmission of nociception include the PVG, medial and lateral hypothalamus, medial preoptic/basal fore-brain region and somatosensory nuclei of the thalamus.

Mesencephalic structures

The PAG receives inputs from the frontal and insular cortex, limbic system, septum, amygdala and hypothalamus. The input from the cortex representing cognition may be involved in activation of the PAG (Basbaum & Fields 1984).

The PAG has ascending projections to the intralaminar nuclei of the thalamus in a pattern similar to that known for the paleospinothalamic tract (Basbaum & Fields 1978, Mancia & Otero-Costas 1973).

Neurochemistry

The PAG contains enkephalin cells and terminals, dynorphin cells, terminals of beta-endorphin axons, substance P, VIP and probably other peptides.

Morphine or the endogenous opioids (enkephalin, dynorphin, beta-endorphin or all three) do not act directly on the PAG output neuron but rather by inhibiting an inhibitory interneuron (Basbaum & Fields 1978). In addition to morphine and the endorphins, the non-opioid peptide sub-stance P produces naloxone-reversible analgesia when injected into the PAG (Lewis et al 1971). Substance P cells are not common in the ventrolateral PAG and dorsal raphe (where there are a large number of enkephalin cells) but there is a high concentration of substance P terminals in this region. It has been suggested that enkephalin neurons probably receive significant substance P input and that this neurotransmitter acts on local opioid peptide neurons.

Rostroventral medulla and pons

These areas receive projections from the PAG and send axons to the spinal cord. In animal studies, electrical stimulation at low intensities of these areas produces analgesia (Basbaum & Fields 1984).

Neurochemistry

The agents and terminals of descending systems that originate in raphe nuclei and medulla are primarily monoaminergic and release serotonin and noradrenaline and less importantly enkephalin and other peptides such as neurotensin.

A number of studies have shown that a descending noradrenaline system appears to be important for opiate-induced analgesia and dorsal horn inhibition and that the noradrenaline descending system appears to be critical for opiate-induced analgesia (Dubner & Bennett 1983). Dysfunction of the ascending noradrenaline system may play a role in pathological anxiety, affective disorders and schizophrenia

Multiple bulbospinal systems

There are many transmitters and pathways involved in bulbospinal modulatory systems (Dubner & Bennett 1983, Le Blanc & Gatipon 1974). Not only are there multiple brain stem sources of axons in the dorsolateral funiculus, but within the rostroventral medulla (RVM) there are cells with different transmitters. Thus there are neurons in the RVM that contain serotonin, substance P, enkephalin, thyrotropin-releasing hormone or almost any combination of the four (Basbaum & Fields 1984). Furthermore, serotonin, substance P and enkephalin are present in RVM cells that project to the spinal cord. In addition to providing separate pathways to the spinal cord, these parallel systems also interact at the brain stem and spinal levels.

Dorsal horn

The interaction between putative primary afferent neurotransmitters and the endogenous opioids existing in dorsal horn interneurons and in terminations of descending inhibitory systems are important for the transmission of nociceptive and other sensory information to the higher centres. This will determine whether information will reach these higher centres and thus whether pain will be experienced. (Hammond 1986, Atweh & Kuhar 1977, Hughes 1975).

DESCENDING FACILITATORY SYSTEM

It has been suggested that there is a bidirectional modulation of nociception. Not only is there an endogenous analgesia system, but the same nuclei and pathways may also contain a specific mechanism for enhancing transmission of nociceptive information. This possibility of bidirectional central control over nociception offers a new explanation for the variability of pain.

Summary

In a study of contributory factors to back pain, an appreciation of the role of biochemical factors is important.

In the early stages of back pain, such as following trauma, endogenous biochemical agents are released and mediate transmission of nociceptive impulses and associated phenomena in response to pain. Neurotransmitters are present at every level of the CNS and are involved not only in pain transmission but also in autonomic, somatovisceral and psychological responses to pain. It is thought that opioids are involved in inhibiting pain and peptides such as SP facilitate pain. The monoamine transmitters are implicated in mood, particularly depression and it is queried whether depressive symptoms commonly experienced by chronic pain patients result from a disturbance in these neurotransmitters.

SUMMARY OF MAIN POINTS

1. Various neurotransmitters and peptides are involved in the production of the experience of pain.

2. Tissue damage caused by injury, disease or inflammation releases endogenous pain-producing substances into the ECF that surrounds the nociceptors. These excite the nociceptors and also alter the local microcirculation and cause hyperalgesia until the injured tissue has healed.

3. There are many types of neurotransmitters in the central terminals of primary afferents. These include the endogenous opioid peptides and non-opioid peptides such as SP.

4. The peptides modulate pain at various levels of the neuraxis. The opioid peptides are thought to have an inhibitory action on pain and have been implicated in the mediation of placebo analgesia. They have also been widely used for the treatment of pain. They play an important role in the descending pain control system.

5. Non-opioid peptides such as SP, VIP, and CCK are thought to facilitate pain and are also involved in somatovisceral and autonomic responses to pain.

6. The monoamines are related to emotional responses and mood. In particular, serotonin has been associated with sleep disturbance and depression.

7. There exists a descending pain control system which consists of four, tiered CNS parts. A number of opioid, non-opioid and monoamine transmitters are involved in this pain system.

8. Neurotransmitters are present at every level of the CNS and are involved not only in pain transmission but also in autonomic, somatovisceral and psychological responses to pain.

4

Modulation of nociceptive input

Nicola Adams

INTRODUCTION

Modulation is the process by which transmission of nociceptive and non-nociceptive information is enhanced (facilitated) or impaired (inhibited), and this is achieved through the interactions of inputs from the periphery, from the interneurons in the neuraxis and from descending control systems from the brain.

These interactions involve endogenous biochemical agents and neural circuitry. This process of modulation determines the character of nociceptive information that is ultimately received by the highest areas of the brain. Thus, the experience of and response to pain are affected by the process of modulation. Treatment to relieve pain aims to modulate the flow of nociceptive impulses to the brain.

Modulation may occur at several levels such as at the periphery, the dorsal horn and at different levels of the higher centres.

An example of peripheral modulation is the action of aspirin, which raises the threshold of peripheral nociceptors (Gilman et al 1991, Rang & Dale 1991). It is the only known example of peripheral modulation of pain, since adaptation only occurs to a very slight extent. All other forms of pain modulation take place within the CNS.

Nociceptive input from the periphery can be enhanced by several factors including:

* sensitization of nociceptors by repeated noxious stimuli
* lowering of the nociceptors' threshold by pain-producing substances
* segmental reflex responses provoked by tissue injury.

Nociceptive input from the periphery can be inhibited by the following:

* Raising the threshold of nociceptors to pain-producing substances, e.g. aspirin.
* Physical treatments such as rubbing or vibration. This may stimulate non-nociceptive large diameter alpha-beta fibres. Stimulating the large diameter fibres may inhibit nociceptive information from the small

diameter fibres. This mechanism has been explained in the theory below. In addition, pain-producing substances which were discussed in the previous chapter may be removed from the area by these techniques as they improve blood flow to the area.

• Electrical stimulation. Electrotherapeutic agents influence the process of modulation in a number of ways. Again they may stimulate the large diameter fibres and they may also assist in the removal of pain-producing substances (Kitchen & Bazin 1996). For a fuller description of pain reduction by electrotherapy, the reader is referred to Kitchen & Bazin 1996.

THEORIES OF PAIN MODULATION

Modulation also takes place within the CNS. To explain the mechanisms of action, an important theory of pain modulation was proposed by Melzack & Wall (1965). This theory has since been updated and suggests a process of modulation known as 'gating', which exists at various levels of the neuraxis.

The gate control theory

The proposed gate consists of small internuncial neurons located within the substantia gelatinosa and a transmitter cell for relay of information to higher levels (Fig. 4.1). Whether or not the transmitter cell is activated is

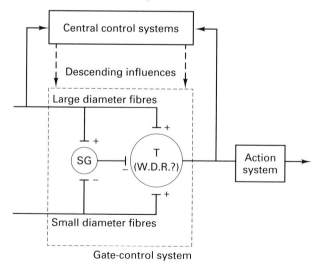

Figure 4.1 The gate control theory of pain. Key: SG = substantia gelatinosa; T = transmitter cell; WDR = wide dynamic range cells; + = excitation; − = inhibition.

determined by a balance between the input of large diameter A-beta and small diameter A-delta and C afferent fibres acting directly through the internuncial neuron.

The gating mechanism can also be influenced by descending influences from a central control system. The theory postulates that small fibre afferent activity would stimulate the transmitter cell, resulting ultimately in the perception of pain. A collateral branch of the small afferent fibre is thought to inhibit the internuncial neuron in the substantia gelatinosa which would reduce the presynaptic inhibitory effect on the transmitter cell. The effect of this disinhibition would be to further enhance trans-mitter cell firing by small fibre input.

Large diameter A-beta fibre input activates the transmitter cell and also stimulates the substantia gelatinosa cell. Since the influence of the SG cell is thought to be inhibitory, increased activity in this cell would counteract the direct facilitatory effect of the large diameter fibres, thus closing the gate and disallowing conduction in the transmitter cell (Echternach 1987, Bowsher 1988, Melzack & Wall 1989, Charman 1989).

An example of the above is 'rubbing a pain better'. When low-threshold mechanoreceptors (A-beta fibres) are activated by rubbing, their collateral endings (which terminate on the terminals of A-delta and C nociceptor fibres in the outer laminae of the spinal cord) partially excite the noci-ceptor terminals. Then, when impulses come along the nociceptor fibres, they find the terminals in a refractory state. The quantity of transmitter substance released from the nociceptor terminals in response to impulses coming along their own fibres is thus reduced. Therefore the gate is 'closed' by the physiological mechanisms of presynaptic inhibition. A-beta fibres appear to have an overall inhibitory gate closure effect on noci-ceptive input and ascending transmission.

Substantia gelatinosa cells and outer dorsal horn cell layers receive a rich innervation from descending corticospinal, reticulospinal, nucleus raphe magnus-spinal and associated tracts. Although the corticospinal tract is normally associated with patterns of voluntary movement activity (Evarts 1975), some 40% of its fibres are sensory afferents from the cerebral cortex (Charman 1989). The fibres may exert gate closure by voluntary distraction of attention away from pain. Thus psychological approaches may reduce the experience of pain through these neurophysiological mechanisms. This is an important concept and is addressed in later chapters.

Criticisms of the gate control theory

This theory is the most satisfactory model of pain theory to date. How-ever, several criticisms of the theory have been made. Nathan (1976) points out that:

1. The proposed properties and functions of transmitter cells are hypothetical, although cells in the dorsal horn of the spinal cord have been found which may exhibit the necessary characteristics.

2. For various pathological states, one should, using the gate control theory, be able to predict whether or not a patient will be in constant pain, or even perceive any pain at all. Thus, selective removal of large fibres should result in all stimuli causing constant pain, and the selective removal of small fibres should result in no stimuli producing any pain. Some conditions, such as post-herpetic neuralgia do not seem to fit this prediction.

There are also various neuropathies with selective destruction of large fibres that do not result in every stimulus producing pain and others showing a decrease in small fibres which does not render the patient immune to pain as would be predicted by the theory.

The updated gate control model has been extended to include modulation at higher levels of the CNS. Probable levels of modulation include not only the dorsal horn but also the brain stem, thalamus and corticolimbic systems. Thus psychological factors exert an effect on neurophysiological input.

LEVELS AT WHICH MODULATION OCCURS

As stated previously, the gate control theory has been updated to include modulation occurring at several levels of the neuraxis. The probable levels at which modulation occurs are at the dorsal horn, brain stem, thalamus, reticular formation and corticolimbic systems. In addition, recent research has implicated the role of the hypothalamus in endocrinological and immunological responses to pain.

Dorsal horn

This is the 'main gate' of limb, trunk and neck sensory input. A combination of peripheral and central descending nociceptor gate control systems interrelate in the SG and outer horn layers.

Intervention at this level may involve reduction or blocking of nociceptive information. This may be achieved by selective activation of large diameter fibres which in turn inhibits the amount of nociceptive information which can pass through the gate. This may be achieved by high-frequency/low-intensity TENS and interferential currents and by manual therapy. In addition, it has been suggested that repetitive high-frequency stimulation at around 100 Hz may produce a physiological block to nociceptive information (Walsh 1991).

Brain stem (medulla, pons, midbrain)

The extensive reticular formation nuclei act as an integrative area where ascending normal sensory and nociceptive collaterals and relays interact with descending higher centre and periaqueductal grey (PAG) input (Williams & Warwick 1980, Chudler & Dong 1995). These interactions involve the integration of psychological factors which neurophysiologically and neurochemically affect the perception of and response to pain.

As discussed in the previous chapter, opioids are involved in the modulation of pain. The PAG is rich in opioid peptides and PAG opioid output is said to be boosted by sharp 'fast pain' sensory stimulation such as some forms of acupuncture and high-intensity TENS (Wolf & Rao 1982).

Thalamus

The groups of thalamic nuclei receive both normal sensory and nociceptive ascending input together with corticolimbic relays. Thus the thalamus also acts as an integrative area in the processing of pain (Talbot et al 1991).

Gating control mechanisms may be analogous to those in the dorsal horn (Charman 1989).

Reticular formation

The RF is a non-specific system. It receives information from all parts of the nervous system and projects back to these regions and modulates their activities through complex mechanisms involving synaptic neurotransmission, autonomic and neuroendocrine effects. The functions of the RF have been discussed in a previous chapter. It exerts influence over pain perception through its projections to thalamic, cortical and subcortical structures (Kenshalo & Willis 1991). These interactions may partly explain the emotional and visceral hormonal reactions to pain and thus the variability of the subjective report of the pain experience.

Cognitive and emotional factors may be used to reduce the intensity of pain via the RF nuclei and this may partly explain analgesia as a result of psychological methods of pain control (Elton et al 1983).

The RF in the brain stem discharges impulses continually and exerts an inhibitory effect on pain by closing the gate in the substantia gelatinosa via the reticulospinal tract. Increasing reticular inhibitory activity will thus decrease the experience of pain.

Reticular activity may be increased by distraction, concentration on another activity, sleep, hypnosis, emotional states that increase blood catecholamines and drugs such as valium and morphine (Wyke 1987). The inhibitory effect is decreased by exposure to sudden intense pain, as this channels attention in the absence of distracting stimuli.

Corticolimbic systems

Cognitive factors such as beliefs, expectations and attitudes towards pain, and emotional factors such as anxiety and depression can enhance or suppress neurochemical and neurophysiological activity in cortical areas and the limbic system. These factors may reduce or magnify the intensity of pain irrespective of its origin.

These areas have considerable input to other areas of the brain, and thus cognitive and emotional activity can exert considerable influence on the perception and response to pain. Addressing cognitive and emotional factors may be used to reduce the experience of pain (Gamsa 1994).

The cortex regulates the activity of the RF by way of corticoreticular fibres and exerts both a facilitatory and inhibitory influence (Kenshalo & Willis 1991).

Variation in the activity of this system may underlie the changes in awareness of peripheral nociceptive stimuli that are associated with alteration in the direction of attention and the induction of hypnosis (Elton et al 1983). Cortical activity is augmented by anxiety, fear and uncertainty and by substances such as caffeine, and thus the experience of pain is magnified. Cortical activity is reduced and reticular activity augmented by emotional tranquillity, sleep and hyperventilation. Hence the experience of pain is reduced.

TREATMENT TO INFLUENCE MODULATION

As modulation may occur at the periphery and also at various levels of the neuraxis, different treatment approaches may be interpreted as influencing the process of modulation at different levels of the neuraxis. Examples of treatment to influence modulation are shown in Table 4.1.

As discussed previously, aspirin may influence peripheral modulation by increasing the threshold of nociceptors to endogenous chemicals produced in response to tissue trauma or ischaemia. Physical treatments, e.g. electrotherapy or manual therapy, influence the process of modulation at dorsal horn level, whereas psychological treatment, e.g. cognitive–behavioural therapy, influences the process of modulation at corticolimbic level (Walsh 1991).

These processes are not viewed apart and separately. Due to the neurophysiological and biochemical interaction discussed in previous chapters, it can be seen that influencing psychological factors will elicit physiological and neurochemical responses. In addition, when giving a primarily physical treatment, the interaction of patient and therapist also affects psychological factors, e.g. providing reassurance, which reduces anxiety. Reducing anxiety, through the interaction of neurochemical and neurophysiological factors mentioned previously, will reduce the experience of

Table 4.1 Levels and treatment to influence modulation

Site of modulation	Example of treatment
Corticolimbic system	Behaviour modification Cognitive strategies Psychotherapy Counselling
Brain stem PAG opioid system	High-intensity TENS Acupuncture Deep acupressure
Reticular activating system	Hypnosis Distraction Diazepam Morphine Chlorpromazine Diaphragmatic breathing
Dorsal horn	Surgery Ultrasound Manual therapy Acupuncture Low-intensity TENS Interferential
Peripheral	NSAIDs Cryotherapy Ultrasound Laser Manipulation Thermotherapy

pain. The implications of these interactions are further discussed in later chapters. From this model, it can be seen that a combined treatment approach should in theory produce the best outcome, as modulation will take place at various levels of the neuraxis.

It should be remembered, however, that pain is often a protective mechanism, especially in the case of acute pain. Thus it is important to manage pain appropriately so that pain is not blocked, e.g. by electrical stimulation, to the extent that the person engages in activity prematurely before damaged tissues have healed.

Conversely, in the case of chronic pain, where pain is limiting recovery, it may be necessary to employ several strategies to modulate pain and encourage activity. This form of treatment is often employed in rehabilitation programmes where patients are taught to manage their pain.

Thus, accurate diagnosis is essential and this is presented in a later chapter.

The model of pain modulation, in addition to offering an explanation for pain reduction, may also provide some explanation of how pain may be maintained beyond peripheral input. If pain transmission can be inhibited, then it can also be facilitated. As a psychological approach can be used to reduce pain, then it follows that psychological factors may also enhance and maintain pain. Thus, psychological approaches and interventions are a major consideration in the treatment of any pain condition.

The following chapters address these psychological factors and also psychological interventions.

Summary

Pain may be modulated at various levels of the neuraxis, including the periphery, dorsal horn and higher centres. Various treatments modulate nociceptive impulses at these levels. In particular, physical treatments affect modulation at dorsal horn levels, and psychological approaches modulate pain at corticolimbic levels. These levels are neurophysiologically and neurochemically interrelated and all exert an effect on each other. The gate control mechanism has been proposed to explain the process of modulation and though it has attracted some criticism, it remains the most satisfactory theory to date.

SUMMARY OF MAIN POINTS

1. Modulation is the process by which transmission of nociceptive and non-nociceptive information is facilitated or inhibited. This is achieved through interaction of inputs from the periphery, neuraxis and from descending control systems from the brain.

2. The gate control theory of pain is the most satisfactory theory to date. It proposes a 'gating' mechanism in the SG of the dorsal horn which can selectively inhibit or facilitate nociceptive impulses. The original model has been updated to include 'gating' at various levels of the neuraxis.

3. Treatments to influence modulation may exert their effects at different levels of the neuraxis, e.g. physical treatments may modulate pain at dorsal horn levels whereas psychological treatments may modulate pain at higher levels.

4. Psychological, neurophysiological and biochemical factors are interrelated and modulating one factor will exert an effect on the others.

5

Psychosocial factors affecting pain

Nicola Adams

INTRODUCTION

The experience of pain is not simply in direct relationship to the amount of peripheral nociceptive input. There are considerable psychological components which affect pain response and these are reviewed in subsequent chapters.

A number of psychosocial variables have been implicated in pain states and may affect perception and response to pain. These include factors such as cultural background and social environment, and people's own beliefs, attitudes and expectations of their pain, the health professional and their treatment.

SOCIAL CONTEXT

The social context in which an injury occurs and hence the meaning of the situation can have a profound influence on a patient's experience of pain and the response to the pain. This was demonstrated by Beecher (1959) who observed the behaviour of soldiers severely injured on the battlefield in the Second World War. These soldiers, in contrast with civilians who had undergone routine surgical procedures, complained of little pain and rarely requested analgesia such as morphine to relieve the pain. Most of the civilians on the other hand requested morphine. The difference in interpretation of the pain was explained in that for the soldiers the battle was over and they had escaped from the battlefield alive whereas for the civilians the pain was an inconvenience and disruption to their everyday lives. Additionally, the military role demands a much greater stoicism, and the social connotations of being a war hero injured (but not killed) in battle are quite different from those of being a person undergoing, e.g., a cholecystectomy. There is also the consideration that soldiers experience guilt at being alive and unharmed when others have been killed or seriously disfigured. Thus, the experience of being seriously enough injured to justifiably leave the battlefield, whilst having done one's duty and risked oneself, means that the soldier does not have to experience feelings of guilt.

This variation in pain tolerance due to the meaning of the situation as attributed by the social context can also be seen in studies of tribal rituals where people insert sharp skewers through their cheeks or dance on hot coals. Such pain is endured for the spiritual reward which is attributed to these acts by the social culture in which they occur. Such attitudes to pain as a 'necessary evil' or as a punishment from God also prevail in western society and will influence people's perception of and response to their pain.

Similarly, the context in which an injury occurs in civilian life will have effects on the patient's interpretation and experience of pain. Otherwise healthy people who are involved in road traffic accidents may rate their pain as more severe than people who have had the opportunity to prepare for their pain, as in the case of elective surgery (French 1992). Patients who are having elective surgery are undergoing this procedure to ameliorate symptoms they have been experiencing and, as such, the surgery and its associated pain is known to be finite, controllable and the outcomes will result in improved quality of life. In the case of the sudden accident, there is great disruption in the normal everyday life of the patient and there are many social implications and uncertainties, e.g. in the case of a man with three children, whose work for a shipping company involves lifting and transporting heavy boxes and furniture and who injures his back in an accident. There are clearly great economic implications and his circumstances are quite different from those of, e.g., a person who is not working and who is financially but perhaps not emotionally supported. In this case the injury has no economic implications but may elicit care and attention which was not perceivably present beforehand. Therefore it is important to assess the impact of psychosocial factors when examining a low back pain patient.

CULTURAL DETERMINANTS

Responses to pain differ not only between individuals but also between cultures. There is much evidence to suggest the existence of differences between nationalities in their expression of pain, e.g. Zborowski (1969) studied the expression of pain in different nationalities. He found that Irish Americans were inhibited in their expression of pain while Italian and Jewish patients were more reactive. The latter two groups drew attention to their pain by expressive behaviour, but the Italians were concerned with obtaining pain relief whereas the Jews wanted to know the cause of their symptoms.

The impact of the social environment is seen in the religious rituals of some cultures, e.g. in Africa, during religious ceremonies, members of certain cults walk on burning coals and insert spikes into their flesh and do not exhibit pain (Weisenberg 1977).

The way in which a child acquires patterns of behaviour about pain is by observational learning (Bandura 1977) and modelling of the pain experience. Children of families who disregard their pain behaviour were found to grow up more stoical in their approach to pain than children who are given undue attention for every minor ailment or complaint. These people may grow up using pain as a way of obtaining attention from others. Thus social modelling within the family groups is a source of individual differences in pain experience (Craig 1978). Parents teach their children ways of avoiding pain and injury, and of discriminating the signs of illness and health, as well as compliance with therapeutic regimes. They also provide positive or negative reinforcement for the display of pain behaviours and emotional and cognitive coping strategies in response to injury.

INTERACTIONS WITH FAMILY MEMBERS

Interactions with family members and family dynamics may have an effect on both the member with chronic pain and the relationships within the family.

Effects of chronic pain on the marital relationship or partner

It has been found repeatedly that chronic pain patients tend to have poor relationships with their partners and show poor sexual adjustment. Ahern & Follick (1985) found that 20% of 117 spouses of patients with chronic pain reported clinically significant symptoms of depression, and over 35% rated their marriages as maladjusted. These marital maladjustment ratings were found to be positively associated with the patients' levels of functional impairment.

However, there appears to be a subgroup of pain patients and partners who share painful symptoms or beliefs regarding pain (Flor et al 1987). Swanson (1984) found some evidence that greater congruence between the attitudes of patients and partners is associated with poorer treatment outcomes.

Effect of family interactions upon patients' pain behaviours

Chronic pain·patients report having more pain patient models in their families than control individuals. Thus observational learning may be related to the development of chronic benign pain or other forms of abnormal illness behaviour. If a family is oversolicitous about minor injuries or ailments, and these are used as a way of receiving attention, it is likely that the individual will respond to such symptoms in a similar manner. Schneider & Wilson (1985) found a high incidence of alcoholism in the families of chronic pain patients and a number of these patients had suffered physical or sexual abuse in childhood.

High levels of spouse reinforcement were associated with high levels of pain and low activity levels. Spouses' reports of reinforcement were also associated with longer duration of pain, high levels of patient satisfaction with marriage and spouses' ratings of:

- high interference of patients' pain with spouses' lives
- positive mood
- high life control.

Thus, partners who tended to reinforce patients' pain behaviours experienced high levels of interference in their lives, but they may also have been rewarded for their actions by positive mood, perceived life control and patients' expressions of marital satisfaction.

It might prove useful early in treatment to identify partners who are especially responsive to patients' displays of pain. These partners may require intensive training to change their reinforcement patterns and yet maintain their positive moods or perceptions of control over their lives.

AGE AND SEX

Age may be an important factor in assessing pain reaction and treatment approach. Weisenberg (1977) and Merskey (1965) found that there is a significant correlation between age and responses to pain. Merskey (1965) found that in a psychiatric population the complaints of persistent pain were most frequent in the older age groups. However, this may be in part explained by the older age groups having greater degenerative processes and thus being likely to have more pain complaints.

Studies assessing sex differences in pain tolerance and response have proved inconclusive. Some studies have shown that there is no difference in pain threshold between males and females, while others have claimed that females have a lower pain tolerance than males (Merskey & Spear 1967). However, there is a difference in the prevalence of the particular pain complaint between the sexes.

FEELINGS OF CONTROL OVER PAIN

Chronic pain patients often feel that their pain has control over them rather than being able to control their pain. Such feelings of loss of control and of hopelessness and helplessness can lead to anxiety and depression, and the experience of pain and concomitant symptoms tends to be magnified.

Cox & Mackay (1982) found that lack of emotional support during crises and inappropriate coping styles were associated with an increase in adrenal cortical activity. (The corticosteroids have been implicated by Selye (1978) in the aetiology of diseases such as ulcers, gastrointestinal upsets and fatigue.) Authors such as McDaniel (1971) and Maas (1972) have carried out studies detailing the effects of cognitive defences, coping strategies and previous experience on the adrenal cortical response. They all concluded that lack or loss of control was an important factor in determining the magnitude of the adrenal cortical response, with an increase in feelings of control over a situation reducing the levels of secretion.

These findings would suggest that a treatment programme to reduce pain and dysfunction should be concerned with developing patients' abilities to manage their pain, rather than become pain victims, by utilizing both physical and psychological methods. Such an approach has been taken by several authors including Williams (1989) who developed a behaviour-modification programme, incorporating physical activity, for chronic pain patients. She maintained that the therapist–patient relationship became a parent–child relationship. Therapists in the Williams programme encouraged patients to take responsibility for their own share of effort and make their own decisions, which changed the normal therapist–patient relationship into an adult-to-adult discussion and agreement. Exercise and activity in a physiotherapy gymnasium was chosen as the medium for the treatment programme. Using this treatment approach, she obtained an 81% success rate in 200 patients, in terms of functional activities and return to work.

Other studies by Harding & C de C Williams (1995) and Rose et al (1995) have successfully used a cognitive–behavioural treatment programme to develop patients' abilities to manage their pain. These programmes involve education, training in coping skills, goal setting, and functional and activity restoration. The programme by Rose et al is presented in a later chapter (p. 152).

PAST EXPERIENCE

Individuals learn how to interpret pain and respond to it by observing others. This means that the role models within the family are of considerable importance to the way in which an individual responds to pain. Thus the individual's past experience of response to pain will affect future responses to it. Similarly, past experience of pain in the clinical setting will influence an individual's response to pain, e.g. people who have had a painful experience on a previous occasion will feel anxious when returning for treatment and this may heighten their experience of any discomfort.

Thus it is important for the therapist to reassure patients and inform them about treatments which may cause discomfort, that they are not harmful and will be beneficial in the long term.

EMOTIONAL STATE

People who are anxious are more sensitive to pain than people who are not (French 1992). This is because cortical activity is increased with a subsequent decrease in reticular inhibitory activity. Thus the 'gate' in the spinal cord is opened to painful stimuli via the reticulospinal tract as discussed in Chapter 4. The intensity of pain has been found to decrease if anxiety is reduced by giving subjects control over the situation. The anticipation of pain, and uncertainty regarding its cause, tend to raise anxiety which in turn increases its perceived intensity. If people understand the cause of their pain, e.g. that the pain is due to part of the lumbar disc pressing on the spinal nerve, they are less likely to be anxious about it and worry that it is due to a spinal tumour. Similarly, pain is better tolerated and probably perceived as less intense if the person believes it to be temporary or 'normal', e.g. pain that is caused by exercise or menstruation.

Anxiety may be relieved and pain reduced by giving patients control, e.g. by allowing them to terminate a procedure at any time if it becomes uncomfortable. Flint (1988) found that familiarity reduces anxiety and advised that the patient be treated by the same professional at each visit if this were possible.

Anxiety may also be reduced by giving patients information about their condition and providing details of their treatment.

Sensitivity to pain is also increased if the person is depressed. This may be due to certain neurotransmitters, e.g. serotonin, in the body which are associated with chronic pain and also depression. It may also be due to the psychological effects of having pain which imposes inactivity, perhaps a loss in work status and limits social activities. The person becomes more focused on the pain and feels increasingly helpless, hopeless and socially alienated and isolated. Depression may be relieved by use of anti-depressant drugs (Blumer & Heilbronn 1982), treating the pain, and the patient feeling in control of the pain with the reassurance and empathy of the practitioner. Thus it is important to involve patients in their treatment programme and provide a feeling of control over their pain. Increasing physical activity has been found to improve mood and self-esteem, and the social contact with the professional has the potential to be therapeutic.

Caution must be exercised, however, for repeated contact with the professional may encourage dependency and focus patients' attention upon their pain. Thus there is a delicate balance between providing treatment and reassurance and allowing patients to take control over their pain.

SOMATIZATION AND PAIN

Most cases of functional low back pain involve somatization not malingering (Capra et al 1985). For these patients, somatization represents an exaggerated fear of re-injury or a way of expressing a repressed fear, anxiety, or depression that has been provoked by one of many real or imagined losses. (This can include subliminal awareness of the loss of function caused by normal or premature ageing.) In general, these patients have spent a lifetime either ignoring the emotional component of their lives or being overwhelmed by that emotional component.

Schneider & Wilson (1985) found a high incidence of alcoholism in the families of chronic pain patients, and often these patients may have histories of alcoholism, smoking and clinical obesity. If patients use these coping mechanisms to avoid depression and anxiety, then it is not unusual that these people will somatize when their emotional life becomes difficult or overwhelming.

As patients recover from chronic disability and their function improves, their rating on scales such as the Oswestry Disability Questionnaire will improve. Basic personality traits as measured by the MMPI tend to show little change, with the exception of the clinical scales of depression, hypochondriasis and hysteria. Beck Depression Inventory (BDI) scores usually decrease. This may be a distinguishing factor between somatizing patients and malingerers, and the latter show little change on these scales.

PATTERNS OF ILLNESS BEHAVIOUR IN CHRONIC PAIN PATIENTS

Chronic pain patients often display abnormal illness behaviour. Pilowsky & Spence (1975b) isolated the following factors of abnormal illness behaviour which chronic pain patients are often found to display:

1. *General factor.* Patients typically experience a phobic concern about their state of health and show interpersonal alienation.

2. *Conviction of disease.* Patients are convinced that they are suffering from a serious illness and the symptoms experienced do not correlate with the physical signs.

3. *Perception of illness.* Patients' perception of the seriousness of their illness is magnified and they report diverse symptoms. Additionally, any minor ailment such as a headache is also magnified and interpreted as a serious symptom.

4. *Affective inhibition.* Patients are restricted in their range of emotional expression and are focused upon their symptoms. It is unclear whether this is in response to pain or whether patients who develop abnormal illness behaviour are poorly socially developed and use their illness as a way of communicating with others.

5. *Acknowledgement of anxiety and depression.* Patients typically experience feelings of anxiety and depression. Often they have experienced these symptoms prior to the onset of their pain (Polatin et al 1993).

6. *Interpersonal and social problems.* These patients tend to form poor social relationships and use their symptoms to attract the attention and care that they crave from those around them. Although they may initially gain sympathy and attention, their continual craving for this in the long term alienates others and thus they become more isolated.

7. *Irritability factor.* Patients often report lowered tolerance and increased irritability associated with their condition and their feelings of anxiety, depression and social isolation.

Health professionals should take these factors into consideration when treating chronic pain patients and employ appropriate communication skills to address the patients' concerns, but without reinforcing abnormal illness behaviour.

ATTITUDES AND BEHAVIOUR OF HEALTH PROFESSIONALS

Health professionals have their own perceptions and ideas of appropriate pain behaviour, based on personal and professional experience. Waddell et al (1984) and Williams (1989) found that patients with low back pain frequently exhibit inappropriate behaviours, and advised therapists not to respond solicitously to these behaviours. It has been found that patients receive maximum sympathy and attention when they exhibit behaviours that are considered appropriate to draw attention to their condition. A low back pain patient who exhibits many pain behaviours and demands much attention from clinical staff is likely to be considered melodramatic, hypochondriacal and difficult, and staff may actually spend less time and attention on this patient than one who is considered a good sufferer. Thus, the complaining patient may exhibit even more bizarre behaviours to attract attention. It is therefore important to reassure patients that they have received the therapist's attention, and that the therapist has understood their problems and is committed to carrying out the most appropriate treatment for them. Once the patient has understood this, it is then considered appropriate not to respond in a dramatic way to exaggerated behaviours. According to French (1992), professionals have considerable power to define and manage pain according to their own attitudes and beliefs.

THE PLACEBO EFFECT

Spiro (1986) defines the placebo as: 'a substance or a procedure that is administered with suggestions that it will modify a symptom or sensation, but which, unknown to the recipient has no specific pharmacological impact on the reaction in question'.

All treatments given by any practitioner can be assumed to contain some placebo element (French 1992). Beecher (1959) found that severe postoperative pain could be relieved in 35% of patients by the administration of a placebo, whereas morphine relieved pain in about 75% of cases. In clinical trials where patients are given either an active drug or a placebo, and given the same explanations, the effects of the drug and placebo tend to be similar. The colours and brand names of drugs have been found to affect the placebo response. Melzack & Wall (1988) found that two placebo capsules are more effective than one, that large capsules are more effective than small ones and that placebos are more effective when given by injection than when administered orally. They also found that placebos become less effective with repeated administration. Spiro (1986) claimed that diagnostic procedures, surgery and the interaction between practitioner and patient all have a powerful placebo effect.

The placebo response varies greatly from one individual to the next and in the same individual from time to time according to the circumstances. Most people are susceptible to varying degrees. As belief in the treatment or the person administering it is central to the placebo response, the effectiveness of specific placebos will be culturally and temporally limited. In western countries, taking placebos in the guise of drugs is likely to be effective. Rachman & Philips (1978) claimed that placebos are more effective in people who are anxious, sociable, conventional and dependable and are least effective in those who are isolated and mistrustful. Melzack & Wall (1988) found that the only consistent difference is that placebo reactors had higher levels of trait anxiety.

Patients' belief in the medicinal value of the treatment does not appear to be crucial. French (1989) cites a study by Park & Covi (1965) in which patients were told that they were receiving medication made of sugar but it was implied strongly that the medication would help. They found that the placebo effect still operated. Thus belief in those administering the treatment is of great importance. This has considerable implications for health professionals. Patients may still find the placebo effect useful even if they are aware of a possible placebo effect, e.g. they may find contact with a health professional helpful even though their condition is not improving. This may be attributed to a feeling of keeping the situation in control.

It is likely that the placebo effect is enhanced or even produced by the degree of understanding, empathy and enthusiasm of the clinicians prescribing or dispensing it as well as their own belief in it. Balint (1964) believes that the clinician can be a more powerful therapeutic agent than the treatment administered and states that it is the social relationship between doctor and patient that engenders this powerful therapeutic effect. Benson & McCallie (1979) reported a 70–90% success rate in response to a placebo in trials conducted by professionals who were enthusiastic about the treatment they advocated. This reduced to a 30–40% success rate when conducted by sceptics. This may also in part explain the popularity and success of the increasing numbers of alternative therapies available, which though lacking in scientific evaluation, are often reported to be effective in alleviating physical and psychological conditions.

The setting in which the treatment is given also has an effect, e.g. a clinical setting where the professional is wearing a uniform and operating technologically advanced equipment, which may all act as representing professionalism and healing, can influence beliefs and expectations of recovery (French 1992). Similarly new or novel treatments such as laser treatment tend to engender higher expectations among patients and increase the placebo response.

Thus the total treatment effect is dependent on the following factors (French 1992):

- the attributes of:
  - the treatment itself
  - the health professional carrying out the treatment
  - the person receiving the treatment
- the setting in which the treatment is administered.

Mediation of the placebo effect

There is still a limited understanding of the placebo effect. The theories listed below are factors that have been considered as mediating the placebo response.

- biochemical effects
- patients'expectations and beliefs
- reduction of anxiety and depression.

It is thought that mediation of the response is brought about primarily by the patients' expectations and beliefs and that these can cause changes in behaviour which can physiologically affect treatment outcomes. In addition, reduction of anxiety and depression can be brought about by reassurance and explanation provided by the therapist and also the effects of the treatment in reducing pain and increasing function. As anxiety and depression are mediated biochemically, it can be considered that the placebo effect has psychological, physiological and biochemical components.

Criticisms of the placebo response

Several criticisms of the placebo response have been made. It is difficult to ascertain whether improvement in a patient's condition is due to the placebo effect (assuming that no treatment was given) or whether this is due to natural resolution of the condition. In addition, there is also the factor of compliance with the clinician, particularly if he or she is making a particular effort, and the patient may report improvement to 'please' the · clinician.

There are also some ethical issues raised by using placebos if the patient is unaware, and the reader is referred to Sim (1989) for fuller discussion of this subject. Nonetheless it can be said that all treatments do have some component of placebo effect and this in part mediates improvement.

PRIMARY, SECONDARY AND TERTIARY GAIN

Primary gain.   The primary gain of any given symptom is the reduction of psychological conflict. Because chronic pain patients are rarely seen in psychoanalytic treatment, the primary gain is not usually clarified. The majority of chronic pain complaints are not directly related to the principle of primary gain. Most chronic pain syndromes originate with minor trauma. From then on, secondary gains can operate.

Secondary gain.   This is defined by the American Psychiatric Association as external gain derived from any illness, such as personal attention and service, monetary gain, disability benefits and release from unpleasant responsibility. Secondary gains are a major aspect of the behavioural theory of chronic pain. Behavioural approaches suggest that pain behaviour is maintained by its reinforcing consequences in the environment, which is a secondary gain. Many aspects of the environment encourage the continuation of pain complaints, e.g. disability benefits, sick leave and litigation awards.

Tertiary gain.   The concept of tertiary gain was introduced by Dansak (1973). Tertiary gain refers to the personal and environmental advantages to persons other than the identified patient in the patient continuing to have pain, e.g. the patient's spouse receiving significant emotional gains from the patient's pain or the family gaining financially or interpersonally from the patient's pain.

IMPLICATIONS FOR PRACTITIONERS

It is important for the clinician to consider these psychosocial factors when assessing the pain patient. Many of these factors will already be addressed in routine clinical interview, such as the age and sex of the patient, the context in which the injury occurred, past history of the pain and previous treatment. In addition, the patient's current functional and working status can be ascertained.

On clinical examination it is usually apparent whether there are abnormal illness behaviours such as exaggerated responses to pain and movement. The emotional state of patients may also be ascertained by their behaviours, e.g. if they are agitated, nervous, tearful or unusually despondent.

This information contributes to the clinician's plans for treatment. However, if the patient exhibits abnormal illness behaviour, this may indicate a poor response to treatment. In this case it may be necessary to determine further psychosocial details such as the effect of the patient's condition on significant others and their response to the patient. Many partners may reinforce illness behaviour by oversolicitous concern or by inconsideration of their partner's condition and thus the patients exhibit further illness behaviours to attract attention to their condition. Often the practitioner can influence outcomes of treatment by giving patients their attention, empathizing and understanding their social problems, and focusing on what can be done to resolve difficulties. It is also important to reinforce well behaviours such as increased function and to increase the patients' feelings of control over their pain by teaching them to manage their pain. (Psychological approaches to treatment are discussed in later chapters.) Thus the attitude and behaviour of practitioners may mediate improvement in addition to their prescribed treatment.

Summary

A number of psychosocial variables may affect the perception of pain and responses to it. These include the social context in which an injury occurs, differences between individuals and between cultures, interactions within families, and age. Studies assessing sex differences in pain tolerance and response have proved inconclusive. Individuals learn how to interpret pain and respond to it by observing others. This means that the role models within the family are of considerable importance to the way in which an individual responds to pain. People who are anxious are more sensitive to pain than those who are not and most cases of functional low back pain involve somatization not malingering.

The response of patients to treatment is influenced both by their own attitudes and behaviours and by those of the health professionals who carry it out. All treatments have some component of placebo effect, which in part mediates improvement, and it is likely that the effect is enhanced or even produced by the degree of understanding, empathy and enthusiasm of clinicians. The setting in which the treatment is given also has an effect.

SUMMARY OF MAIN POINTS

1. Many psychosocial factors have been found to affect a person's perception of and response to pain. These include factors such as social background and environment and people's own beliefs, attitudes and expectations of their pain, the professional and their treatment.

2. Factors such as social modelling and interaction with family members are important in assessing whether pain behaviours are reinforced in the social environment.

3. Emotional factors such as anxiety, state of mind and past experience all affect perception of the experience and response to pain.

4. The interaction of the patient and practitioner may have a powerful therapeutic effect and the attitudes and behaviours of health professionals influence a patient's response to treatment.

5. Several theories have been considered as mediating the placebo response including both psychological and biochemical explanations.

6

Psychological models of chronic pain

Nicola Adams   Douglas Taylor

INTRODUCTION

Psychological factors play an important role in acute and chronic pain (Gamsa 1994, Klaber-Moffett & Richardson 1995). A number of psychological models have been proposed to explain why pain may progress to become chronic, and psychological treatment approaches have been based on these models (Rose et al 1995).

In this chapter, the psychological models that have been proposed in chronic pain are presented. These models address different mechanisms as determinants of chronic pain. No one model has been determined to be superior to the other models, and so all are considered.

Exploring psychological factors which have been implicated in chronic pain through these models may provide an indication of psychological characteristics of low back pain patients who develop chronic pain, and treatment approaches have been based on these models.

The models of chronic pain which have been proposed are:

1. psychodynamic/personality models, e.g. Engel (1959)
2. behavioural models, e.g. Fordyce et al (1968)

Table 6.1 Major models of chronic pain

Type of model	Theory	Contribution	Limitations
Psychodynamic/personality	Emotional and personality characteristics involved in the development of pain	Recognizes psychosocial variables Explains individual variability	Methodological restraints in research
Behavioural	Pain behaviours are learned and reinforced	Methodological improvements in pain research	No consideration of individual response style or coping skills Do not offer model or cause of pain
Cognitive–behavioural	Relationships between cognitive processes and mood on behaviour	Recognizes complexity of pain experience	Do not offer model of cause of pain Possibility of mixed messages Difficulty in evaluation
Psychophysiological	Interaction of physiological and psychological factors in pain	Control of autonomic and physiological responses to pain	Lack of correlation with subjective pain report

3. cognitive models, e.g. Turk et al (1983). In Table 6.1 these are subsumed under cognitive–behavioural models.
4. cognitive–behavioural models, e.g. Turner & Romano (1990)
5. psychophysiological models, e.g. Middaugh & Kee (1987).

The models are summarized in Table 6.1.

PSYCHODYNAMIC/PERSONALITY MODELS

The theory underlying these models is that emotional factors may generate and perpetuate chronic pain (Engel 1959), and emotional difficulties may be expressed as pain (Shanfield & Killingsworth 1977). The authors suggest that certain types of personality may predispose to the development of pain from organic lesions. Alternatively, another theory is that organic lesions causing pain may promote the emotional and personality changes (Woodforde & Merskey 1972).

Schneider & Wilson (1985) argued that all disease is psychosomatic in origin, with some diseases having more emotional aspects than others. They further suggested that disease results from environmental factors such as diet, climate and a deeply conditioned belief system which precludes the ability of the brain/mind to respond adaptively to environmental stimuli. Bellack et al (1982) suggested that this inability to respond adaptively to external stimuli may have resulted from early parental conditioning, psychosocial factors and perceptual factors.

Whatever approach is taken, it is clear that psychological factors are involved in the pain experience whether the pain has an organic basis or is disproportional to the objective clinical signs and symptoms. It is the extent to which they contribute to the pain experience that is variable from one individual to the next.

The psychosocial variables which have been examined for their aetiological significance include personality traits such as depression (Bradley et al 1993, Klapow et al 1993, Ahles et al 1987), hypochondriasis (Pilowsky 1970), anxiety and obsessionality (Harper & Steger 1978, Collet et al 1986) and family dynamics (France et al 1986).

The following section aims to explore personality factors involved in the chronic low back pain syndrome. The major personality characteristics that have been implicated in chronic pain patients will be presented in this chapter.

Certain symptoms of emotional disturbance are more characteristic of patients who have relatively little evidence of physical findings. Such patients tend to score higher on the psychological scales of depression, hypochondriasis and hysteria, often with a peak at depression (Carron & McLaughlin, 1982 Finneson 1980, McCreary et al 1980). Patients who do not have a clear organic pathology have been found to rate their pain as more intense and as high in terms of affective and evaluative descriptions on the McGill Pain Questionnaire as compared with patients with organic pathology.

The principal dimensions of personality and emotional disturbance that typify chronic low back pain patients are listed below. Some of these dimensions identify patients who are at high risk for poor response to standard medical treatments.

DIMENSIONS OF PERSONALITY DYSFUNCTION

It was found by Shanfield & Killingsworth (1977) that personality dysfunction could be described in terms of the following dimensions:

- a dimension of emotional disturbance that reflects interpersonal alienation and distrust, but this did not differ from the normal population to any significant degree
- somatic concern, which was clearly differentiated from the normal population, showing elevated hypochondriasis and hysteria
- a dimension that involves vulnerability, openness to admitting problems and a perceived lack of control over life circumstances

- a dimension that reflected extroversion and social desirability.

The dimension of emotional disturbance that did predict good versus poor outcome from conservative medical treatment was somatic concern.

EMOTIONAL FACTORS IN HEADACHES

Muscle contraction headaches and low back pain have been found to be related to emotional and psychological stress (Main 1992, Waddell 1987). Headache sufferers have shown increases in the psychasthenia, depression, hypochondriasis, hysteria and anxiety scales on psychometric testing as compared with a population without pain. Such patients report feelings of inadequacy, obsessive–compulsive behaviours, indecision and worry, depression, anxiety, paranoid feelings and cognitive confusion. Measures of pain frequency have been found to be related to the depression, hypochondriasis and hysteria scales (Harper & Steger 1978) and measures of subjective pain have been found to correlate significantly with physical complaints and illness frequency.

PERSONALITY PROFILE OF BACK PAIN PATIENTS

Patterns of skeletal muscle participation in the behaviour of 65 subjects with low back pain were studied by Holmes & Wolff (1952) in an attempt to evaluate a personality profile of patients exhibiting the backache syndrome. It was found that there was increased motor and electrical activity of skeletal muscle in response to situations which threatened subjects' security and engendered apprehension, conflict, anxiety and feelings of resentment, hostility, humiliation, frustration and guilt. Such subjects are often unable to give expression to their hostile feelings, having an excessive need for praise and approval, becoming petulant and demanding or angry in their attempts to extract sympathy and support from those upon whom they are dependent for their security. As adults they substitute an agggressive, self-assertive, outgoing and intensely competitive pattern of behaviour. Others, as children, had attempted to protect their sensitive feelings and gain approval by being well behaved and quick to comply with demands made of them, with little or no attempts at overt expression of hostility. As adults they become shy, submissive and withdrawn non-participators. Both types are basically immature, insecure, sensitive and excessively dependent on their action 'patterns' for protection against the many threats to their security, often being neat, meticulous and perfectionistic. These observations were consistent with those of Wilson (1990) in his profile of the neuromuscular responder to stressful situations.

More recent research has found variable results in testing low back pain patients for EMG activity, though it has been uniformly demonstrated that LBP patients show a higher overall EMG activity and higher skin conductance than pain-free subjects, which is suggestive of autonomic arousal.

Physiologically, relatively intense and sustained skeletal muscle activity in response to either physical trauma or emotional disturbance, leads to vasoconstriction and spasm in muscle which may progress to myofascial pain syndromes and changes in the pathology and function of that muscle. Ischaemic changes and the increased metabolism of the muscle with decreased oxygen supply leads to a change in the biochemical environment of the muscle with a gradual accumulation of noxious tissue metabolites which may perpetuate nociception. Therefore the physiological response may be initiated by psychological factors, and the response progresses in the same manner whatever the nature of the initiating factor.

Leavitt & Garron (1980) found that low back pain was related to inhibition of aggression and hostility, and that low self-esteem distinguished these patients in the Tennessee Self-Concept Scale, whereas Spengler (1980) suggested that a guilt-ridden, self-punishing personality is one of the initial causes of intractable pain. He postulated that physical pain may restore an individual's self-esteem by allowing him to believe that he would be capable of succeeding in all areas were it not for his physical affliction. Prokop & Bradley (1980) reported that many low back pain patients experience unmet dependency needs early in life which are not gratified until a physical injury provides a socially accepted means of depending on others for emotional and economic support. These people learn to live with their pain by deriving satisfaction from their role as invalids.

From previous studies, it would appear that the characteristics of depression, somatization of mental conflicts and somatic concern are important psychological components of the chronic pain syndrome.

PERSONALITY FACTORS INVOLVED IN BACK PAIN

There is general agreement among authors that personality factors involved in back pain include:

1. depression
2. hypochondriasis (somatic concern)
3. conversion disorder (hysteria)
4. anxiety
5. obsessive–compulsive behaviours, general maladjustment (psychasthenia), lack of cognitive flexibility
6. neuroticism and social introversion.

Depression

Definition

Jayson (1981) described depression as an excessively sad mood without obvious cause or disproportional to the problem.

Types of depression

Depression is commonly described as being either:

- vegetative (endogenous) (Carron & McLaughlin 1982), where sleeping, eating and sexual functions are affected, or
- reactive, which is generally secondary to chronic pain or other external factors.

Depression may be 'masked', that is a depressive disorder may be underlying a principal somatic complaint (Lopez Ibor 1972, Forrest & Wolkind 1974). Masked depression may be either reactive or endogenous.

Lopez Ibor (1972) stated that one in four or five cases of depression consult a psychiatrist. He also observed that there are three fundamental groups of clinical symptoms in which depression may be masked. These were:

1. Pains and paraesthesias, e.g. headaches, pain in the scapular and lumbar regions.
2. Psychosomatic disturbance. Kreitman & Sainsbury (1965) observed that depressive patients with somatic complaints had a greater tendency to develop psychosomatic disorders.
3. Changes in sleeping and eating patterns.

Chronic pain and depression

One reason for the ability of pain to mask affect and affective disorders is that, as Sternbach (1986) has noted, chronic pain is similar in its signs to depression in that the physiological, behavioural and affective effects of chronic pain and depression are quite similar. Patients who are suffering chronic pain (of whatever cause) typically report loss of appetite, sleep disturbances, decreased libido, inability to concentrate, loss of ability to function at work, low self-esteem, feelings of hopelessness and helplessness and a general apathy and lethargy. These self-reported symptoms are similar to those patients suffering from depression would report to a clinical psychologist or psychiatrist.

Models of chronic pain and depression

While a substantial body of literature does show that patients tend to be depressed (e.g. Romano & Turner 1985, Adams et al 1994), mechanisms linking pain to depression are not well understood (Doan & Wadden 1989).

Although depression is viewed as a personality characteristic, several models are proposed to explain its occurrence in chronic pain. They include:

- cognitive–behavioural model (Rudy et al 1988)
- biochemical model (Ward & Bloom 1982)
- dysthymic pain disorder (Blumer & Heilbronn 1982).

Cognitive–behavioural model. (This model is discussed in more detail on p. 86.) Rudy et al (1988) proposed a cognitive–behavioral model of chronic pain and depression based on the results of 127 chronic pain patients. They proposed that perceived reduction in activities of general living (ADL) along with a decline in perceptions of control and personal mastery are necessary prerequisites for the development of depressive symptomatology in pain patients. They found no direct link between pain and depression but found that perceived interference and self–control were intervening psychological variables.

Biochemical model. Ward & Bloom (1982) proposed a biochemical model of chronic pain, based on treatment studies on relieving pain by the use of antidepressants, that similar neurochemical mechanisms involving catecholamines, serotonin and endogenous opioids contributed to both depressive disorders and chronic pain. They proposed that adrenocortical secretions result in a higher intracellular sodium content in depression, thereby causing fluid retention and swelling of the intervertebral discs, with their possible protrusion. Almay et al (1988) compared healthy volunteers with chronic pain patients and patients with definable neurogenic pain syndromes for depressive symptomatology, personality characteristics and the results of a series of biochemical tests. It was found possible to discriminate among the chronic pain patients, the healthy control group and the definable neurogenic pain syndrome group on the basis of measurements of 5-hydroxyindoleacetic acid (a metabolite of serotonin) before and after dexamethasone suppression, and melatonin in serum and urine. This implicates the role of serotonin in depression.

Dysthymic pain disorder. The theory of dysthymic pain disorder proposed by Blumer & Heilbronn (1982) based on the evaluation of 2000 patients with chronic pain, viewed chronic pain as the principal expression of an underlying depressive disorder. Patients with dysthymic pain were found to share certain biological characteristics with patients suffering from major depression. While abnormally shortened rapid eye movement is found to a lesser degree in the dysthymic patients, abnormal sleep efficiency is at a very high level in both groups. Ahles et al (1987), in a study of 45 primary fibromyalgia syndrome (PFS) patients, 29 rheumatoid arthritis (RA) patients and 31 non-pain controls, found no difference between PFS and RA groups using the Zung Self-Rating Depression Scale, though they did not use a biochemical test. They concluded that the hypothesis of the presentation of chronic pain in the absence of known organic pathology as a variant in depressive disease was not supported in the case of PFS. The authors conceded, however, that a sub-group of PFS

(28.6%) and RA (31%) patients appeared to be experiencing significant depressive symptomatology.

Factors predicting treatment response

Dworkin et al (1986), in a study of 454 chronic pain patients, 79 of whom were classified by the Diagnostic and Statistical Manual of Mental Diseases (DSM-III) scale to be depressed, found in predicting treatment response, that in non-depressed patients a number of factors were important. A beneficial response to treatment was related to factors such as:

- a greater number of treatment visits
- not receiving compensation
- fewer previous episodes of treatment and incidences of low back pain.

In the case of depressed patients, a better response to treatment was found if the patient was in employment and had pain of shorter duration.

These results suggest that activity and active involvement in treatment are particularly important for depressed low back pain patients.

It was found by Forrest & Wolkind (1974) that there are distinct populations of patients with low back pain. The 'poor' response group was characterized by a depressive syndrome described principally in somatic terms ('masked'). The MMPI thus demonstrated an ability to predict response to treatment. It may therefore play a part in the further investigation of patients not responding to conventional treatment. Leavitt & Garron (1980) using the Back Pain Classification Scale (BPCS) against the MMPI, correctly identified 87% of the sufferers of low back pain and whether the pain was of an organic or functional nature.

Populations of chronic pain patients

A study by Klapow et al (1993) has indicated, using cluster analysis on results obtained using the McGill Pain Questionnaire (MPQ), Sickness Impact Profile and Beck Depression Inventory, that there are three groups of chronic pain patients:

- chronic pain syndrome—this group was characterized by high levels of pain, high levels of impairment and high levels of depression
- positive adaptation to pain—this group was characterized by high levels of pain but low levels of impairment and depression
- good pain control—this group was characterized by low levels of pain, impairment and depression.

This study shows the effect of depression as a variable affecting patients' reports of the level of their pain and impairment. Forrest & Wolkind (1974) in agreement with these findings found distinct populations of patients with low back pain where the poor response group was characterized by a high level of depression and somatic symptoms.

Hypochondriasis and somatic concern

Definition

Bellack et al (1982) described hypochondriasis as the unrealistic fear of disease, having such characteristics as anxiety, depression and compulsive personality traits.

Somatic concern is a category of hypochondriasis.

Types of hypochondriasis

Carron & McLaughlin (1982) described two types of hypochondriacal patients, based on the relative passive–dependence or overt hostility present. The passive–dependent patient has an excessive dependence on the medical staff, complying with all instructions, whereas the 'masochistic–hostile' hypochondriac is more persistent and may demand referral to a specialist and specialized investigations.

Finneson (1980) lists physical signs associated with hypochondriasis, e.g. bizarre reactions to drugs, nervousness, irritability and tension headaches. Kreitman & Sainsbury (1965) observed that marital disharmony, poor sexual adjustment, incidences of childhood abuse and poor parental relationships and the chronicity of illness were common features in the case histories of these patients. When tested against a normal population, they were described as more habitually anxious and worried than the control group. It was also found by Kreitman & Sainsbury (1965) that hypochondriasis tends to be reactive to an event or illness rather than an endogenous characteristic.

Mayou (1991) found hypochondriasis to be a significant factor in patients presenting with medically unexplained physical symptoms, in agreement with Pilowsky & Spence (1976) and Marbach et al (1983) who found significant correlations between illness behaviour and pain estimate in myofascial face and back pain patients. These findings would suggest an increased somatic concern in chronic pain patients; however, it must be considered that the effect of pain as a stressor affecting autonomic and neuroendocrine systems results in various physiological somatic responses (Main 1992).

Sainsbury (1960) determined six characteristics that may function as complicating psychological factors for patients with chronic low back pain, on the basis of an orthopaedic examination of 36 low back pain patients, but did not provide information as to the age and sex of the patients or the pathology of their pain. These characteristics were:

- vague history of past illness
- resentment and criticism of physicians

- dramatic symptoms and their reactions to them
- difficulty in localizing and describing pain
- failure of usual treatment to give significant relief
- accompanying neurotic symptoms.

Conversion disorder

(Conversion disorder was previously known as hysteria.)

Definition

Conversion disorder is a complex and difficult topic both conceptually and clinically. Crown (1978) described conversion hysteria as the translation of a mental conflict, for example anger or sexuality, into a somatic disturbance in the sensorimotor systems which has no acceptable organic basis and which is potentially reversible (e.g. by suggestion, hypnosis or psychotherapy).

Carron & McLaughlin (1982) described cases where recurrent and multiple somatic complaints developed an actual somatic problem. This somatization could then lead to a conversion or somatoform disorder (Sternbach 1986). Conversion disorder implies a loss or alteration in physical functioning, suggestive most often of a neurological, endocrinological or autonomic dysfunction. While the symptoms are not consciously produced, the patients, none the less, achieve primary gain such as anxiety reduction as well as secondary gains such as compensation or favourable attention from their spouse and other environmental supports as a result of them (Caldwell & Chase 1977). If pain alone is the presenting complaint, psychogenic pain disorder rather than conversion is diagnosed. To be correctly diagnosed as a conversion disorder, the disturbances in physical functioning of the presenting condition cannot be explained by a known physical or pathophysiological disorder and usually appears to provide some reward in the patient's life.

Blumer & Heilbronn (1982) in describing the characteristics of dysthymic pain disorder would appear to be describing the characteristics of hysteria as defined by the previous authors. It has been found by McCreary et al (1979) that chronic back pain patients score highly on the depression and hysteria scales on the MMPI, with hypochondriasis, although elevated for the pain groups, not as high as on the other two scales. It may therefore be postulated that there is an interrelationship between hysteria and depression.

Chronic pain patients have difficulty in expressing their feelings to other people (Pilowsky & Spence 1976). Alexithymia is a common finding in psychosomatic and addictive disorders where the emotions tend to be undifferentiated and poorly verbalized and most are experienced in the somatic sphere. Individuals with alexithymia may appear stoic, expression-less and posturally rigid (Ahreus & Deffner 1986). They are oriented towards physical work and mechanical action and they lack imagination and fantasy. Crown (1978) suggested that neurophysiologically, alexithymics may lack neuronal connections between the limbic system and the neocortex. Therefore drive arousal tends to be expressed through the autonomic nervous system (ANS), neuroendocrine or neuromuscular systems. This view has since been supported empirically by Wilson (1990) in psychophysiological stress profile studies.

Four main personality profiles were isolated by Sternbach (1986) using the MMPI on such patients. These were:

- neurotic depression
- hypochondriasis
- hysteria and conversion reactions
- elevated psychopathic and hypomanic scales.

Woodforde & Merskey (1972) argued that there is a close relationship between chronic pain and hysteria rather than depression, and associated the hysterical personality with low socioeconomic status and psychogenic sexual disorders. Contrastingly, both Wolkind (1974) and Finneson (1980) refer to 'la belle indifference' in hysterical patients, where lack of appro-priate distress in the face of severe complaint is encountered.

Anxiety

There are many definitions of anxiety, as the term is often used with different meanings. Simpson (1980) defined anxiety as:
A personality characteristic of responding to certain situations with a stress syndrome of responses. Anxiety states are then a function of the situations that evoke them and the individual personality that is prone to stress.

There is a distinction between anxiety as an emotional state and as a relatively stable personality state. These are referred to as trait anxiety, which is a characteristic of the individual, and state anxiety, which is associated with a particular situation. Generalized anxiety disorder (GAD) is described by the American Psychiatric Association (1987) as a relatively persistent, chronic condition of tension implying an enduring and trans-situational trait of the individual. Other categories such as social phobia or post-traumatic stress disorder are classifications in which anxiety is a relatively transient and/or situationally specific response.

France et al (1986) found a high incidence of family alcoholism in chronic pain patients and Krishnan et al (1985), in a study of 71 chronic low back pain patients using a modified Anxiety Scale, found symptoms of anxiety in patients with major depression. It was found that anxious mood, tension and general somatic symptoms were more common than other anxiety symptoms and the authors suggested a treatment programme utilizing relaxation-based biofeedback to reduce anxiety.

The crises of anxiety are often accompanied by a series of symptoms which are projections of these crises on to the somatic and visceral planes. Once the critical phase has passed, the vegetative symptoms also become automatic and independent, and constitute vicious cycles.

Wilkinson (1983) described palpitations, headaches and indigestion as physical manifestations of anxiety. Other psychological factors in anxiety such as resentment, frustration and paranoia and repression of emotions may be translated into physical symptoms (Copeman 1969). His observations were validated by EMG studies carried out by Holmes & Wolff (1952) who described a response pattern involving the musculature in relation to some interpersonal or social situation not being met.

Obsessive–compulsive behaviours and other characteristics

Other factors that have been found to be involved in chronic low back pain include a dimension that assesses anxiety, obsessive–compulsive behaviour and general maladjustment. The MMPI psychasthenia scale incorporates these characteristics. Individuals who score highly on this scale are seen as tense, worried, preoccupied and phobic and they tend to intellectualize and ruminate about problems (Goldstein & Hersen 1984). The high scorer is compulsive and worries about trifling rituals, engaging in repetitive checkings and countings. The highest scores on this scale have been found in alcoholics (Cattell 1973). In the obsessive–compulsive reactions, anxiety is associated with preoccupation with unwanted ideas (obsession) with persistent impulses to repeat certain acts over and over (compulsion). These persons have feelings of helplessness, inadequacy and self-doubts (Wolman 1965).

They tend to be workaholics and exhibit excessive concern with conformity and are rigid, overinhibited, overconscientious, overdutiful and unable to relax easily (Ullman & Krasner 1975). In addition, Miller & Cooper (1988) found the obsessive personality to be a methodical, moralistic personality, meticulous in dress and speech, paying much attention to detail and often having problems making decisions.

The person with a compulsive personality disorder was found to have an inability to express warm and tender emotions and an inappropriate preoccupation with trivial rules and details.

It appears that the genesis of obsessive–compulsive disorders is influenced by a multiplicity of factors, possibly including a genetic predisposition, social learning as mediated by parental modelling and parental control in childhood and various life stresses and learning experiences.

Repressed memories, desires and conflicts are held to be the source of neurotic anxiety which manifests itself as various symptoms.

Collet et al (1986) found a significantly higher level of psychasthenia using the MMPI in patients with tension headaches as compared with a non-pain group. Harper & Steger (1978), in agreement with these findings, found a higher level of obsessive–compulsive behaviour, anxiety, depression, indecision, thought and worry, as determined by the MMPI, in patients with tension headaches as compared with a non-pain group.

Neuroticism and social introversion

Neuroses, or non-psychotic mental disorders are strategies of perception and behaviour which are exaggerated. They are characterized by pathological increases in anxiety and rigid defence mechanisms which are maladaptive. Neurotic people are anxious, fearful, depressed and generally unhappy. They do not suffer from delusions or severely disordered thought processes. Their strategies for coping with life events and stresses are disordered and maladaptive. They tend to avoid rather than confront these stresses and frequently suffer from hypochondriasis and fatigue, and thus overdepend on these maladaptive strategies. The American Diagnostic and Statistical Manual of Mental Disorders (DSM-IV) (American Psychiatric Association 1987), does not use the term neurosis but in its place are the anxiety disorders, somatoform and dissociative disorders and dysthymic disorder. These include GAD, obsessive–compulsive disorder, phobic disorder, conversion disorder and hypochondriasis.

Eysenck & Eysenck (1975) introduced the dimension of introversion/ extraversion, where the introverted person had a tendency to be quiet, retiring, introspective, reserved, serious, reliable and dislikes excitement. Neuroticism and social introversion have been found to correlate closely.

Trait anxiety has been found to correlate with neuroticism. Gray (1985) found that individuals with high trait anxiety possessed characteristics which reflected a combination of introversion and neuroticism. These findings are consistent with those of Bradley et al (1993) and Sainsbury (1960) who reported higher levels of neuroticism, anxiety, social introversion and lack of openness in chronic back pain patients as compared with non-pain populations.

It can be seen that the term neuroticism is merely a general term that embraces a number of characteristics.

CRITICISMS OF THE PSYCHODYNAMIC/PERSONALITY MODEL

The major contribution of these models is that they recognize the individuality of patients and that past experiences, family dynamics and personality characteristics all play a part in a patient's perception and response to pain.

While some of these factors, particularly depression, are appreciated as being important in chronic pain, not only by proponents of the theory but also by proponents of cognitive–behaviourism (Keefe & Dunsmore 1992a and b), the major criticism of these models is the implication that the psychological dysfunction is the aetiological factor in developing pain and that physiological/organic factors are secondary. A study by Polatin et al (1993) found that there was an equal division of depressive symptoms before and after onset of pain in a group of 200 patients with chronic low back pain. As most cases of back pain begin with minor trauma and associated emotional factors (Kirkaldy-Willis 1988) and then progress through various stages of pathology before becoming chronic, it is more helpful to view this model in terms of emotional factors contributing to the pain experience and response rather than being their cause. While psychoanalysis is therefore unlikely to be helpful in treating the majority of cases of low back pain, an important contribution of this model is that it recognizes psychological factors in pain and also their variability from one patient to another.

Overall, the evidence for these models has been inconclusive because results of studies are inconsistent and the methodology is not always sufficiently rigorous due to the emphasis on individual subject variation. However, the plethora of studies investigating psychological and psycho-social variables in pain have determined that emotional and personality factors do indeed affect the experience and response to subjective pain (Polatin et al 1993, Klaber-Moffett & Richardson 1995).

BEHAVIOURAL MODEL

In response to the subjectivity of the psychodynamic/personality models, Fordyce et al (1968) suggested that observations should be restricted to pain behaviours. Behaviour theory defines pain by the presence of 'pain behaviours' (Fordyce 1976, 1986). These are verbal and nonverbal signs of distress that are independent of subjective report. Using an operant learning theory framework, Fordyce postulated that a pain problem becomes chronic because the pain behaviour is positively reinforced while well behaviour is not reinforced. However, the question of what the patient is actually experiencing is avoided in this model (Gamsa 1994).

Respondent pain is defined by Fordyce as a response to continuing nociceptive input within the organism. Operant (learned) pain is a response that has been shaped and moulded by its reinforcing consequences in the environment. Operant pain is maintained because it elicits secondary gain such as permission to avoid chores, unpleasant sexual activity or aversive interaction with family members. Operant pain may also serve to control family members and to obtain otherwise unattainable attention and care. This was supported by Gil et al (1988) who found that higher levels of reported satisfaction with social support correlated with more pain behaviour.

Pain often begins as a response to trauma that causes tissue damage. What happens to the person with acute pain determines whether the pain takes on operant characteristics. Fordyce considered that there are three sets of conditions by which respondent pain may lead to operant pain:

1. Pain behaviours receive direct and positive reinforcement.

2. Pain behaviours receive indirect but positive reinforcement leading to relief of normal responsibilities or successful avoidance of unpleasant circumstances.

3. Activity or well behaviour efforts are negatively reinforced or punished. Linton & Gotestam (1985) showed that in the laboratory setting, pain behaviours may be increased through positive reinforcement and reduced if they are ignored and well behaviours reinforced (Fordyce et al 1973).

To understand pain behaviour in this behavioral framework it is important to ascertain what the consequences of the pain behaviour were in the past and the reinforcers currently operating in the environment which are maintaining pain behaviour. The important components from a behavioural analysis perspective are:

- current activity levels
- pain patterns
- pain behaviour
- medication usage
- interaction with family members.

The high prevalence of pain and illness in family members of pain patients has been cited as evidence for the influence of pain models (Turk et al 1987). Additionally, the concept of observational learning ('modelling') has been used to interpret results of studies which show that members of a family often share similar types and/or sites of pain (Turk & Flor 1983). Family members may learn pain-generating physiological responses from each other, e.g. Block (1981) showed that spouses of chronic pain patients responded with elevated physiological arousal when observing their spouses in pain, which supports a view of observational learning promoting organ system vulnerability.

From this operant perspective, some aspects of pain behaviour are iatrogenically caused by the health care system, e.g. medication use. In the past, pain medication was usually prescribed as the patient 'needed' (wanted) it. This may lead to a learned or conditioned link between pain and medication. Because strong analgesia, such as the narcotic analgesics, have subtle mind-altering effects as well as relieving the pain, medication becomes a reward for the pain.

Another example is the advice given by professionals to rest and not overdo things, which is often part of a conservative management programme. Whilst this is often appropriate for an acute pain patient, there is a risk of a conditioned link between pain expression and inactivity. The problem is defining when acute management should end and more active, rehabilitative efforts should begin.

The appropriate treatment of a chronic pain patient based on behavioural principles requires that pain behaviours are unrewarded and well, normal or healthy behaviours are positively reinforced (Keefe & Lefebvre 1994).

Although it may be possible to reduce pain behaviours by controlling their reinforcers in the laboratory (or in pain management programmes), this is considerably more difficult in the patient's own environment where there may be difficult family dynamics, and interpersonal and social problems. This is also a major criticism of comparing experimentally induced laboratory pain with clinical pain. Pain behaviours are believed to be instrumental in the development of avoidance of activity, which then also becomes a pain behaviour (Fordyce 1976, Waddell & Turk 1992), and consequently may be potent indicators of risk for chronic pain development (Linton 1994).

Main et al (1992) found that scores on a non-organic signs test evaluating some specific 'inappropriate' pain behaviours in the clinic increased with the amount of failed treatment (Waddell et al 1984). However, Bradish et al (1988) found no correlation between the non-organic signs and activity levels 1 year later.

CRITICISMS OF THE BEHAVIOURAL MODEL

The major criticism of this approach is its simplistic interpretation and lack of attention to individual response styles or coping skills.

In response to these criticisms, Fordyce (1979) presented a revised behavioural model of pain behaviour that extended the operant model to take into account the influence of biological and psychological variables. Recent research based on this model has attempted to determine the relative importance of somatic, behavioural and psychological factors in explaining pain behaviour in different chronic pain populations (Keefe et al 1984, 1986).

In summary, behavioural treatment specialists recognize that pain behaviour patterns are learned. Understanding the history of these behaviours, both of early childhood and more recent experiences, is crucial to attempts to change pain behaviour. If behavioural treatment is to be effective, a careful analysis of historical influences on pain behaviour is essential (Fordyce 1976, Keefe & Lefebvre 1994). According to Keefe & Dunsmore (1992a and b), many authors have attempted to reduce the complexity of chronic pain by applying the pain behaviour concept in an overly simplistic pattern and not taken account of psychosocial factors. It can therefore be argued that the original proponents of the theory did not foresee a pure operant model being applied to a variable patient population.

An important contribution of the behaviourists to studies of pain was the introduction of methodological improvements, including carefully designed control procedures and laboratory methods (Gamsa 1994).

COGNITIVE MODEL

Cognitive theory examines constructs such as expectations and beliefs about pain, personal control, problem-solving abilities and coping skills (Gamsa 1994).

The cognitive model, in contrast to the behavioural model, makes a clear statement about the relationships between cognition, affect and behaviour. Cognitive models are often subsumed under the cognitive–behavioural model, as cognitive processes and behaviour are intricately linked.

The assumption of the cognitive model is that cognitive activity is the sole determinant of pain behaviours and/or emotional distress. That is, an individual's emotional distress or behavioural difficulty is not a direct reaction to an untoward life event but rather a direct consequence of how that event is perceived.

Cognitive treatment and assessment involves identifying those dysfunctional thought processes and irrational beliefs that lead to emotional distress and which increase pain perception and experience. Cognitive interventions to control pain attempt to increase the patients self-efficacy, i.e. ability to cope with the problem (Bandura 1977), and are modelled on research which demonstrated that a subject's appraisal of a difficult situation and beliefs about his or her ability to cope with it influence the experience of stress (Bandura 1977). Ciccone & Grzesiak (1984) identified cognitive events which amplify the pain syndrome to include catastrophizing, overgeneralization, low frustration tolerance, external locus of control and mislabelling of somatic sensations.

Thus the focus of the cognitive approach to treatment is on changing the way that individuals think about their pain.

Cognitive theory has added an important dimension to psychological research into pain; however, the influence of mental processes is only part of a complex problem (Gamsa 1994). Turk et al (1983), who themselves use cognitive concepts, do not provide the solution. While successful outcome has been reported in laboratory studies into the effect of cognitive manipulation on experimentally induced pain, results have not been consistent. Turk et al (1983) attribute these inconsistencies to the use of different designs and procedures among studies. More importantly, these outcomes cannot readily be transferred to the clinical situation where an infinite amount of variables exist.

COGNITIVE–BEHAVIOURAL MODEL

The cognitive–behavioural model is essentially a unifying theory, in which the behavioural model is expanded to incorporate cognition and affect within behaviour therapy. It draws upon such areas as behaviourism, social learning theory and cognitive psychology (Grzesiak & Perrine 1987). A variety of psychological interventions are combined within this framework and it emphasizes education, control by the patient and coping strategies. Treatments are usually a combination of cognitive and behavioural interventions such as biofeedback, relaxation training, acquisition of coping skills and operant conditioning (Turner & Romano 1990).

Cognitive–behavioural approaches, like the behavioural approach, do not offer a model of the causes of the pain. However, they do explain how chronic pain can be made worse or maintained by psychological factors. Both assessment and treatment are highly individualized, based on each patient's pain behaviours, conceptualization of the pain problem and ability to cope with the stresses related to pain. Conceptual systems are composed of the following (Turk et al 1983):

- values, beliefs and goals regarding health, disease and illness
- information about the disease and sense of perceived competence
- role expectations and sets of action plans for responding to situational demands.

Pain is viewed as a stressor itself.

The cognitive–behavioural perspective emphasizes the complex interactions between cognition, affect and behaviour. Thus this model views the way in which an individual reacts to pain as a complex, multidimensional response.

Cognitive–behavioural approaches have been used extensively in pain programmes (Weisenberg 1989, Turk & Rudy 1991, Harding & C de C Williams 1995) with some success (Nicholas et al 1992). Main (1992) concluded that there are difficulties in overall evaluation of pain management programmes due to factors such as heterogeneity of the programmes themselves, differences in patient characteristics and assessment instruments, differing outcome appraisal and socioeconomic influences on outcome.

CRITICISMS OF THE COGNITIVE–BEHAVIOURAL MODEL

A major criticism of using cognitive–behavioural treatments is that the potential exists to provide mixed messages about the nature of the pain problem. Ciccone & Grzesiak (1984) indicated that if a patient is receiving a comprehensive treatment programme that includes operant conditioning, biofeedback and coping skills training, then they are being told by the operant philosophy that the environment is maintaining the pain behaviour. However, assumptions inherent in biofeedback and coping skills training are that the individual can modify and self-regulate aspects of the pain problem. Therefore the patient is receiving two opposing messages about the nature of the pain and its control.

On the other hand, if, as will be suggested later, the most effective use of the different models is to combine them into a multimodal strategy using the appropriate components of each, then it will be necessary to give the patient mixed messages. This may in fact, be appropriate. If pain and its treatment can only be described accurately in terms of a combination of different factors from different models, then effective treatment will also necessarily be multimodal.

PSYCHOPHYSIOLOGICAL MODELS

These models consider the interaction of physiological and psychological factors in the development of chronic pain. Psychophysiological studies examine the influence of mental events (thoughts, memories and emotions) on physical changes which produce pain (Gamsa 1994). The possible role of physical responses such as muscle activity, vascular changes or autonomic arousal have been studied extensively in relation to pain disorders such as headaches (Andrasik & Holroyd 1980), myofascial pain and low back pain (Flor et al 1991, Arena et al 1991) with inconsistent findings (Gamsa 1994).

In explaining the mechanisms which link abnormal psychophysiological patterns with pain, two general models are proposed. First, general arousal models propose that frequent or prolonged arousal of the autonomic nervous system, including prolonged muscle contraction, generate and perpetuate pain. In contrast, specificity models explain the development of specific types or sites of pain in relation to individual differences in psychophysiological responding to environmental stressors, due to genetic predisposition, previous experiences and personality type

(Schneider & Wilson 1985). The mechanisms involved, however, are not well understood.

Many individuals demonstrate a distinct physiological pattern in response to a stressor. These response patterns vary from individual to individual and the proponents of the theory postulate that the response patterns determine the type of disease the individual would be prone to develop. The interpretation of what constitutes a stressor is variable and specific to the individual (Cox 1981). Pain may be considered to be a stressor agent and therefore the effects of pain are not only the sensation resulting from the neurophysiological mechanisms involved, but also a complex interaction on every bodily system through nervous and endocrine mediation. This more complete picture of the mechanism of pain may help explain the often diverse symptomatology of the chronic pain complainer.

In order to appreciate these factors, it is necessary to understand the mechanism involved in the reaction to a stressor and the effects on the individual.

ANATOMICAL AND PHYSIOLOGICAL BASIS FOR THE STRESS RESPONSE

The stress mechanism affects every system via nervous and endocrine pathways. It can be set in motion by damaging physical and emotional stimuli (Appley & Trumbull 1986).

The response to stress is both psychological and physiological. The physiological response is dominated by the major psychoendocrine systems, the sympathetic-adrenomedullary and the pituitary– adrenocortical systems (Ganong 1989). This response may occur at one specific site as in the case of local injury or it may be more widespread as in the case of generalized pain (Selye 1978).

Because of the diversity of the functions of the hypothalamus and the functions of the organs which affect and effect the stress mechanism, it can be seen that there will be widespread autonomic and endocrine effects in response to a stressor such as pain (Main 1992). This may in part explain the diverse symptoms reported by pain patients, such as fatigue and gastrointestinal upsets, and may additionally explain the increased levels of somatic concern (hypochondriasis) found on psychological testing of these patients (Main 1992).

Christie & Mellett (1981) found that psychological factors can set off a profound physiological response. In particular, they observed that physiological responses to anxiety conditions included an increase in heart rate, sweating and musculoskeletal pain. In contrast, the physiological responses in patients with depression were found to be reduced cardiovascular reactivity and a low non-reactive electrodermal response. In addition,

Ursin et al (1978) found a suppression of testosterone in response to fear. This may in part explain the decrease in libido reported by depressed and chronic pain patients. Sternbach (1986) found that these patients had characteristically high somatic concern and fear of underlying malignancy, dependency and invalidity.

Mason (1971) suggested that the primary mediator for hormonal release may be the psychological factors involved in emotional or arousal reactions to threatening and unpleasant events in life situations.

Patterns of stress response have been identified by Sternbach (1986) and Schneider & Wilson (1985) using electromyography (EMG), galvanic skin response (GSR), thermal biofeedback and electroencephalography (EEG). They identified the particular response an individual produced in response to psychological stress. These included:

- neuromuscular response
- parasympathetic/depressive response
- neurovascular response
- neurohumoral and neuroimmune response
- interneuronal response.

PATTERNS OF STRESS RESPONSE

Neuromuscular response

In the neuromuscular response style, individuals showed a general tightening of the voluntary muscles during stressful situations. They often presented with tension headaches, and chronic neck and/or low back pain which often progressed throughout the body. The alpha and gamma motor systems controlling voluntary muscle activity are therefore affected in this response.

The difference between this response and other forms of stress response is that tense individuals are often less aware of high skeletal motor activity until pain and spasm are already present. They have a higher baseline of muscle activity which makes them more prone to physical causes of muscle pain, e.g. cold, posture and the effects of injuries and deformities.

Psychologically, it has been observed by Schneider & Wilson (1985) that this type of responder had a high incidence of childhood trauma; in a study of 100 patients, they found that 70% were the adult children of alcoholics and 40% had experienced physical or sexual abuse in child-hood. Most had been children of hypercritical parents who would rarely give unconditional approval.

Thus, the combined effect of psychological and physical trauma produced the disorder of chronic muscle pain in the individuals who respond to stress by bracing their skeletal musculature.

Parasympathetic/depressive response

In the parasympathetic/depressive response style, individuals exhibited a lack of normal physiological arousal levels, rather than an activation of the sympathetic nervous system. The primary conflict in this response pattern appears to be concerned with the blocking and suppression of feelings. Feelings are 'shut down' as a protective reaction to prevent further psychological trauma, when individuals cannot psychologically remove themselves from the situation, e.g. in bereavement. This pattern involves muscular flaccidity or wasting, obesity, blood pressure problems and reduced cardiovascular reactivity. The immune system fails and risks of infection and cancer increase. This response style may arise through stress exhaustion or learned helplessness as a pattern of hopelessness emerges (Seligman 1975).

Although the mechanism is unclear, it is known that the hypothalamus/pituitary alters the production of ACTH in prolonged depression. ACTH stimulates the production of cortisol by the adrenal glands and cortisol in turn suppresses the immune system.

Depressive distress is marked by dry skin and a low, non-reactive electrodermal response. Other glandular functions fail and this may lead to poor digestion, impotence, infertility and/or menstrual problems and thyroid problems (Baker 1987, Christie & Mellett 1986).

Neurovascular response

In the neurovascular stress response, individuals were found to respond to stress primarily with the heart or blood vessels or peripheral neurovascular control mechanisms and may have eventually developed a myocardial infarction, cerebrovascular accident, migraine, Raynaud's disease or premenstrual syndrome (Friedman & Rosenman 1974). These authors described neurovascular responders as having a Type A personality, which is characterized by inner rage, anger, hostility and excessive time consciousness.

Neurohumoral/neuroimmune response

In this response, individuals were found to display an inappropriate endocrine and exocrine glandular coordination and may have developed allergies, or intestinal or reproductive disorders (Schneider & Wilson 1985).

Interneuronal response

In this response, individuals expressed their response psychologically rather than by somatizing and may have eventually developed schizophrenia or manic depressive illness, and they experienced intra-psychic conflict (Karasu & Bellack 1980, Bellack et al 1982). A person may not exhibit one type of response exclusively, but may exhibit a number of these responses to a greater or lesser degree. It appears from the findings of the above authors that there are certain personality characteristics and family histories that are involved in a person's response to stress.

TREATMENTS BASED UPON THE PSYCHOPHYSIOLOGICAL MODEL

Treatments such as static EMG biofeedback and relaxation techniques are designed to reduce levels of muscle activity and autonomic arousal and thereby reduce pain. Such treatments have been shown to be effective in reducing the pain of muscle contraction headache (Andrasik & Holroyd 1980), migraine and back pain, although not necessarily more so than other psychophysiological interventions (Gamsa 1994).

Recent developments in dynamic paraspinal EMG monitoring and bio-feedback have extended these concepts to include correction of dynamic muscular activity (Middaugh & Kee 1987, Cram 1990) with consequent reduction in subjective pain report and increased function (Donaldson & Donaldson 1990, Adams et al 1993).

CRITICISMS OF PSYCHOPHYSIOLOGICAL MODELS

The value of these models has been that they have shown that it may be possible to control the autonomic and physiological responses to pain. However, physiological response has not been shown to correlate closely to subjective pain report. The lack of correlation between physiological state and subjective assessment of physiological state has been demon-strated (Taylor & Lee 1991). In terms of perception of pain, this lack of correlation may be due to an individual's psychological state, needs and expectations and may not reflect the ineffectiveness of strategy in controlling the physiological component of the pain.

INTEGRATION OF THE MODELS IN PRACTICE

Theories of chronic pain have evolved from several schools of thought based upon psychological theories, empirical research and clinical obser-vation. While treatment approaches are based upon these models, they need not be applied exclusively according to one particular model. As stated previously, the cognitive–behavioural model, which in itself combines two major models, is used successfully in pain management programmes (Harding & C de C Williams 1995). It is argued that any patient–practitioner interaction involves a psychological discourse which is based upon a number of variables including the patients' beliefs and expectations, personality, family circumstances and behaviours in addition to their biomechanical or organic dysfunction.

The most effective use of the different models is to combine them into a multimodal strategy using the appropriate components of each model. If pain and its treatment can only be described accurately in terms of a combination of different factors from different models, then effective treatment will also be necessarily multimodal. It is important for patients to understand possible explanations for a disorder as well as possible forms of treatment, so they can assist the practitioner to define what would be the most effective protocol for them given their needs, beliefs and expectations.

Additionally, whether patients are given to understand that it is the environment which is maintaining their pain, or that they themselves are maintaining it, the control of the pain is always given to the patients, not to the environment, even when a behavioural model is emphasized.

IMPLICATIONS FOR PRACTITIONERS

The interaction between practitioner and patient affects psychological factors and may in itself be a mediator for improvement irrespective of the form of treatment (Adams et al 1994). The past experience of patients, social factors and personality factors are considered by practitioners in their assessment of patients and also in devising an appropriate treatment programme, e.g. it is unlikely that anxious patients will respond favourably to a dynamic, highly technological, impersonal approach on their first treatment.

The aims of chronic back pain management programmes include (Harding & Williams 1995):

- improving levels of physical fitness, spinal mobility and posture and thus increasing ability to perform functional activities
- improving the ability to manage stress and improving sleeping patterns
- changing counterproductive beliefs about pain and improving general mood
- reducing the effect of pain on the family and improving social relationships
- teaching effective self-management and maintenance of gains
- reducing dependency on drugs.

These aims may be achieved in several ways:

- explanation and education
- reinforcement and encouragement

- relaxation
- reassurance and reduction of anxiety and depression
- changing behaviour
- distraction.

Explanation and education

Giving an explanation of the cause of the pain makes patients aware of possible reasons for their pain and the aims and reasonable expectations of their pain management programme. There are many lay beliefs about back pain, and patients often receive conflicting and inaccurate advice from unqualified practitioners. Once patients understand basic anatomical and physiological principles of the low back and biomechanical implications of various postures and mechanical stresses, it is then possible to apply these to their daily activities. Modification of posture and lifting activities often results in a significant decrease in pain report. In giving exercises and advice, the therapist is educating patients to manage their pain. If sufficient explanation has been given, patients then understand the purpose of these exercises and are more likely to comply with the instructions.

These strategies may be viewed as having a cognitive–behavioural component.

Reinforcement and encouragement

Reinforcing well behaviours may be viewed from a behavioural perspective and the therapist may also use cognitive strategies to allow patients to reinterpret their pain. Pain may be interpreted as a temporary discomfort from carrying out prescribed exercises, due to stretching little-used muscles and ligaments, rather than as a serious symptom. Patients are encouraged to participate in well behaviours such as increased functional activity and not reinforced for behaviours such as exaggerated facial expression of pain and staggering. This may also improve social relationships as exaggerated pain behaviours and focusing on pain are often counterproductive in obtaining attention and sympathy; these behaviours are often irritating to friends, relatives and indeed health professionals.

It is important that patients also receive encouragement for their efforts and gains. This may be achieved by setting goals for the patient to achieve and maintain.

Relaxation

The use of relaxation techniques to reduce muscle activity is employing a psychophysiological model. Not only does relaxation have a physiological effect, but it also has a beneficial psychological effect and allows patients to reflect more realistically and positively upon their condition. Thus they learn to become less anxious about minor symptoms. Relaxation may also improve sleep patterns, which are often disturbed in chronic pain patients.

Reassurance and reduction of anxiety and depression

Reassurance given to the patient may reduce anxiety, and reducing feelings of hopelessness and helplessness may reduce depression (Seligman 1975). Explaining the general reasons for back pain and making clear that patients' concerns are valid but their fears of serious underlying pathology are usually unfounded will reduce feelings of anxiety or fear. It is often helpful to reassure patients that it is usual to feel low in mood and angry and frustrated about their condition, but that the condition can be improved with resultant improvement in mood. According to Seligman (1975), increasing a feeling of control over the situation and reducing these feelings of hopelessness and helplessness may, in fact, reduce depressive symptoms which are common in chronic pain patients (Polatin et al 1993).

Changing behaviour

As stated previously, it is important to reinforce well behaviours and not to respond oversolicitously to exaggerated staggering and grimacing. Patients often avoid activity for fear of the consequences of activity, i.e. they may do more damage and therefore suffer more pain. Patients are therefore encouraged to participate in controlled activity and thus increase their function.

Distraction

It is often helpful for the therapist to engage in non-task comments while carrying out a painful procedure, as diverting attention can reduce the experience of pain. This technique is commonly used by nurses and doctors while taking blood. Such social interaction also reduces anxiety associated with a highly technologically advanced environment.

It is important that practitioners remain flexible in their approach to treatment and use the psychological models to assist diagnosis and management rather than be constrained by them. Not only is there considerable variation from one patient to the next, but there is considerable variation in the initial and final stages of treatment in the same individual, e.g. patients who attended on the first visit clearly anxious and distressed may require considerable reassurance and explanation in the early stages of treatment, but as their pain decreases and function increases, the anxiety and depression may lessen and the focus of treatment then becomes increasing the patients' control and management of their condition. It is possible for the practitioner to adopt and adapt components from each of the psychological models of chronic pain for the maximum benefit of the patient in this process.

If working in a team involving a clinical psychologist, other professionals should be aware of the psychological approach being employed, so that all members of the team can work together to reinforce this approach.

Specific techniques used in psychological management based upon these models are presented in Chapter 8.

Summary

A number of psychological models—psychodynamic/personality, behavioural, cognitive, cognitive–behavioural and psychophysiological–have been proposed to explain why pain may progress to become chronic. Psychological treatment approaches have been based on these models, but none has been proved to be superior to the others; each has its strengths and its limitations, and all are open to criticism.

It would be inappropriate to apply any one of these models exclusively to psychological aspects of patient management as there are many variables involved in the experience of pain. It is necessary for the reflective practitioner to adopt and adapt components of these models and integrate them into practice.

SUMMARY OF MAIN POINTS

1. The psychological models of chronic pain that have been proposed are the psychodynamic/personality, behavioural, cognitive, cognitive–behavioural and psychophysiological models. Each has its strengths and limitations.

2. According to the psychodynamic/personality model, emotional factors may generate and perpetuate chronic pain. Psychosocial variables which have been examined for their aetiological significance include personality factors and family dynamics.

3. The personality characteristics that have been implicated in chronic pain include depression, hypochondriasis, conversion disorder, neuroticism and social introversion, anxiety and obsessive–compulsive behaviours.

4. Behavioural theory defines pain by the presence of 'pain behaviours'. Using an operant learning framework, it is postulated that these behaviours are learned and treatment based on behavioural principles requires that the contingencies are reversed so that pain behaviours are unrewarded and well behaviours are positively reinforced.

5. The cognitive model makes a relationship between cognition, affect and behaviour. The assumption is that cognitive activity is the sole determinant of aberrant behaviour and/or emotional distress, i.e. an

individual's emotional distress or behavioural difficulty is not a direct reaction to an untoward life event but rather a direct consequence of how that event is perceived.

6. In the cognitive–behavioural model, the behavioural model is expanded to incorporate cognition and affect within behaviour therapy.

7. Psychophysiological models consider the interaction of physiological and psychological factors in the development of chronic pain.

8. It is possible to adopt and adapt components from each of the psychological models of chronic pain in treatment programmes.

7

Assessment

Nicola Adams   Douglas Taylor

INTRODUCTION

In this chapter methods for assessing the low back pain patient will be detailed. These will include:

1. measurement of pain
2. methods for psychological assessment
3. physical methods of assessment
4. electromyographic assessment
5. assessment of function and disability.

An accurate diagnosis is essential prior to devising an appropriate treatment programme. This should include psychological testing, physical examination and assessment of functional activity.

A complete assessment of low back pain should include the following tests as this information is important in order to make a correct diagnosis. Many of these tests would be too time-consuming for routine clinical examination and an abbreviated examination for routine clinical use is provided at the end of the chapter.

THE CLINICAL INTERVIEW AND ASSESSMENT OF PAIN

History of the present condition

An accurate history should be obtained to determine chronicity of the condition as the longer a patient has had the pain, the longer it will take to treat. At this time it is important to determine whether the pain may be related to a specific event or whether it is of insidious origin. If the pain is of insidious origin, it is likely to be due to degenerative changes. Often the onset of pain is associated with a specific task carried out in a particular position such as when twisting or lifting. This may result in muscular and articular damage. Pain starts immediately or within a few hours. The number of episodes of pain that the patient has had and any previous treatment should be recorded. This will determine if the pain is of a recurrent or chronic nature and what treatments have been helpful or unhelpful in the past.

Psychosocial factors

Questioning about psychosocial factors may provide useful information in addition to the information obtained from clinical history taking, as psychosocial factors may be important in the response to and per-petuation of pain.

Psychosocial factors to consider are (Capra et al 1985):

- patient and family history related to personal losses and chronic illness
- potential signs of depression
- patient and family mental health history
- any stressful changes in lifestyle or marital status before or since the injury
- financial history, contrasting current income with past income and comparing these with current cost of living
- work history, including explanation of job losses and job changes
- any litigation that is pending for the patient's current medical problem.

Present condition

The current condition should be ascertained to determine the patients current pain status. This will determine whether the pain is present at rest or whether it occurs on movement or at night. This will assist diagnosis. Pain that occurs on movement is usually of biomechanical origin. Pain that awakens the patient at night, which is not associated with movement, or is present unremittingly all day with no variation should be viewed seriously and onward referral to a physician or surgeon is recommended.

Relevant past medical history

This should be considered to determine whether the patient has had a history of serious illness, what investigations have been carried out, etc.

It should be determined whether the patient has had previous lumbar surgery or spinal fracture. No matter how successful symptomatically, spinal surgery in itself produces scarring and impairment and there is similar impairment with spinal fractures no matter how well healed these may be. Therefore these patients will not be expected to return to full function.

Mandatory questions

These questions should include whether the patient has any family history of osteoarthritis or rheumatoid arthritis or any other serious illness such as diabetes or epilepsy. The patient's current medication should be recorded as some drugs and conditions may be a contraindication to some treatment modalities, e.g. a patient with osteoporosis should not be treated with traction or violent manipulation. For contraindications to electrotherapy, the reader is referred to Forster & Palastanga (1981).

X-ray reports may be useful to determine whether the patient has existing degenerative changes, an old spinal fracture or spondylolisthesis.

Patients who have a severe nerve root prolapse, metabolic disorder or other serious organic illness should be treated by a physician or surgeon.

PAIN

Pain is difficult to measure as it is a subjective experience. It also has sensory, affective and behavioural dimensions.

The sensory aspect of pain is probably the easiest to assess. This relates to the location and qualitative nature of the pain, whether it is sharp or a dull ache, where it occurs and its intensity, e.g. the pain in the lower left side of the back and it aches.

It should be determined whether pain is the patient's main problem or whether the main problem is loss of function. The site of pain should be recorded on a body chart and the nature of the pain described as this will assist diagnosis, e.g. a dull ache is indicative of degenerative changes and OA which will require treatment to relieve pain and increase blood flow to the area. On the other hand, a sharp pain on movement may be indicative of muscle or joint disorders which will require a different type of treatment.

Duration and frequency

Acute biomechanical LBP usually lasts for a few days ranging to 12 weeks. In about 7.1% of cases, pain may become chronic. Pain of myalgic origin is usually relieved within 1 week and disc herniations may require 8 weeks to resolve. Disc degeneration may cause chronic discomfort that is exacerbated during acute attacks which can last for a few weeks. Mechanical pain tends to be intermittent in nature and tends to be associated with exposure to mechanical stresses. Pain that is constant and never varies is usually of medical origin. Spinal tumours cause persistent pain that builds in intensity over time.

Location and radiation

Most mechanical causes of back pain are localized to the lumbosacral region. Damage or degenerative change in the lumbar disc or facet joints may cause referred pain in the buttock and thigh. Pain that radiates to the lower leg is suggestive of nerve root involvement and also may indicate a trigger point with referred pain in the piriformis muscle (Travell & Simons 1983, Taylor 1990). Sacroiliac involvement may also cause pain in the lower back with or without radiation.

Aggravating and alleviating factors

Biomechanical lesions improve with rest and are worsened by prolonged sitting, lifting or twisting. Prolonged inactivity may also worsen biomechanical back pain and may lead to chronicity as pathological changes occur in underused or inappropriately used muscles. Bed rest for several days is advised for muscle strain; however, it has not been shown to be helpful beyond this time period. Back pain that is non-biomechanical, i.e. is due to other medical pathology, is worsened by rest.

Time of day

Pain due to biomechanical disorders is usually worse at night as the patient has been up and around all day. Patients with arthritic conditions, fibromyalgia or those with concomitant depressive symptoms tend to be worse in the morning, due to poor sleep and stiffness associated with immobility. Patients with spinal tumours have most pain at and during the night. The risk of disc herniation is greatest in the morning due to the fluid content of the intervertebral discs being greatest at this time.

Measurement of pain

Pain intensity is most directly evaluated by patient reporting. Although electrophysiological techniques for sensory evaluation exist, including nerve conduction studies, EEG, somatosensory evoked potential monitoring and microneurography, each has its own technical difficulties in interpretation. These techniques have proved to be useful in assessing experimentally induced pain. However, there are important differences in the evaluation of experimentally induced pain as compared with acute and chronic clinical pain. The difference between clinical pain and experimental pain lies in the emotional and cognitive factors which are important in the experience of clinical pain. Psychological factors may greatly influence pain perception and experience. Experimental pain focuses almost exclusively on the sensory aspect of pain, removing the affective and sociobehavioural variables which are involved in clinical pain.

The sensory dimension of pain is most often quantified in linear fashion. Linear scales can be discontinuous 'ordinal' scales which contain descriptive words (such as 'mild', 'moderate' and 'severe' pain) or they may be a continuous representation such as the visual analogue scale (VAS).

Ordinal scales (Waddell 1987)

The therapist may make an assessment of pain based on a simple grading.

1. *Mild.* Pain of this degree does not contribute to physical impairment.
2. *Moderate.* Evidence of a pathological state of the involved structures that would reasonably produce pain of the reported level.
3 *Severe.* Pathological changes and clinical findings indicate that physical function is limited by pain which requires treatment for relief.

Visual analogue scale

This is a 10-cm horizontal or vertical line representing a linear spectrum of pain intensity. The opposite ends are labelled 'no pain' and 'worst possible pain.' The patient is asked to make a mark at a point along the line which represents the intensity of pain on this scale. This is simple to administer and score and most patients find it relatively easy to complete. It is often helpful to ask the patients to mark the scale twice, once to represent their usual pain and again to represent their worst pain. Waddell (1987) suggests the use of a vertical VAS in the form of a pain 'thermometer' as illustrated in Figure 7.1.

The major difficulty lies in interpreting exactly what the pain scale measures. It is a subjective measure and often bears no correlation to any physical or pathological change. Thus it is difficult to assess whether the

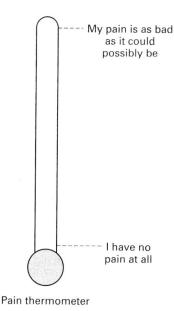

Please put mark on the
thermometer to show how bad
your usual pain is these days

My pain is as bad
as it could
possibly be

I have no
pain at all

Pain thermometer

Figure 7.1   Visual analogue scale.

scale is measuring pain or distress as both are closely interlinked in the clinical setting. It is, however, useful in obtaining an assessment of overall pain intensity as experienced by the patient.

McGill Pain Questionnaire

Quality of pain is frequently assessed by asking the patient to select from a list of descriptive adjectives which best characterizes the pain, e.g. the McGill Pain Questionnaire (MPQ) (Fig. 7.2). This was compiled from a list of adjectives that characterized pain with regard to its sensory, affective and evaluative attributes. The sensory properties of pain have previously been discussed. The affective properties of pain are those qualities which elicit an emotional response from the patient, e.g. fear or anger. The evaluative aspect of pain correlates with pain intensity, but additionally reflects the patient's level of tolerance of the pain experience. The MPQ thus purports to measure the pain experience.

When relating these dimensions of pain to the neurophysiology of pain which was presented in Chapter 2, it can be seen that the VAS, MPQ and psychological scales are in fact all measuring different dimensions of the

McGill Pain Questionnaire

Patient's Name _____ Date _____ Time_____am/pm

PRI: S _____ A _____ E _____ M _____ PRI(T) _____ PPI ____
(1-10)   (11-15)   (16)   (17-20)   (1-20)

1 FLICKERING __
  QUIVERING __
  PULSING __
  THROBBING __
  BEATING __
  POUNDING __

2 JUMPING __
  FLASHING __
  SHOOTING __

3 PRICKING __
  BORING __
  DRILLING __
  STABBING __
  LANCINATING __

4 SHARP __
  CUTTING __
  LACERATING __

5 PINCHING __
  PRESSING __
  GNAWING __
  CRAMPING __
  CRUSHING __

6 TUGGING __
  PULLING __
  WRENCHING __

7 HOT __
  BURNING __
  SCALDING __
  SEARING __

8 TINGLING __
  ITCHY __
  SMARTING __
  STINGING __

9 DULL __
  SORE __
  HURTING __
  ACHING __
  HEAVY __

10 TENDER __
  TAUT __
  RASPING __
  SPLITTING __

11 TIRING __
  EXHAUSTING __

12 SICKENING __
  SUFFOCATING __

13 FEARFUL __
  FRIGHTFUL __
  TERRIFYING __

14 PUNISHING __
  GRUELLING __
  CRUEL __
  VICIOUS __
  KILLING __

15 WRETCHED __
  BLINDING __

16 ANNOYING __
  TROUBLESOME __
  MISERABLE __
  INTENSE __
  UNBEARABLE __

17 SPREADING __
  RADIATING __
  PENETRATING __
  PIERCING __

18 TIGHT __
  NUMB __
  DRAWING __
  SQUEEZING __
  TEARING __

19 COOL __
  COLD __
  FREEZING __

20 NAGGING __
  NAUSEATING __
  AGONIZING __
  DREADFUL __
  TORTURING __

PPI
0 NO PAIN __
1 MILD __
2 DISCOMFORTING __
3 DISTRESSING __
4 HORRIBLE __
5 EXCRUCIATING __

BRIEF __ | RHYTHMIC __ | CONTINUOUS __
MOMENTARY __ | PERIODIC __ | STEADY __
TRANSIENT __ | INTERMITTENT __ | CONSTANT __

E = EXTERNAL
I = INTERNAL

COMMENTS:

Figure 7.2 McGill Pain Questionnaire. (Reproduced with kind permission from Melzack & Wall 1989.)

experience of pain as the ascending nociceptive pathways are conveyed through the various projections of the thalamic nociceptive dispersal system to the different areas of the brain that are involved in the various aspects of the pain experience.

Thus it is unwise to select only one of these measures and it is helpful in clinically assessing the low back pain patient to rate pain on a VAS. If the patient's condition is chronic, it may be helpful to administer a short psychological questionnaire to assess depressive symptoms. Information about the quality and nature of the pain may be easily obtained from the initial clinical assessment.

In a research trial it is possible to carry out a more complete assessment of the patient including use of the MPQ and other psychological scales.

METHODS OF PSYCHOLOGICAL ASSESSMENT

A number of psychological factors have been implicated in the analysis of pain conditions and have been discussed in earlier chapters. Many of these have been subject to psychometric assessment. A psychometric test may be useful to evaluate psychological and personality factors and the extent of their involvement in pain conditions.

When pain, physical impairment and disability are all proportionate, then together they provide a good measure of clinical severity. However, when there is significant disproportion between the patient's report of pain, disability and work loss, the clinicians assessment of the underlying pathology and objective physical impairment, then a more comprehensive assessment is required of the cognitive, affective and behavioural dimensions of the illness.

There are a number of psychometric tests available and the common ones are presented below. The selection of a test is concerned with what the clinician seeks to evaluate. Recent research in back pain has employed questionnaires to assess functional capacity rather than focusing on psychological aspects alone. Many of these questionnaires incorporate a psychological component.

Psychological tests used in the assessment of back pain include:

- Minnesota Multiphasic Personality Inventory (MMPI)
- Modified Somatic Perception Questionnaire (MSPQ)
- Beck Depression Inventory (BDI)
- Illness Behaviour Questionnaire (IBQ)
- Back Pain Classification Scale (BPCS) and Revised Symptoms Checklist SCL-90R)
- Coping Strategies Questionnaire (CSQ)
- Distress and Risk Assessment (DRAM)

- Fear Avoidance Beliefs Questionnaire
- other tests.

Minnesota Multiphasic Personality Inventory (MMPI)

The Minnesota Multiphasic Personality Inventory (MMPI) is a commonly used test delineating the psychological involvement in various medical syndromes. It is designed to assess objectively the various personality characteristics that affect adjustment and integration of an individual, both personally and socially, into society. Nine scales were originally developed for clinical use of the inventory. These were:

- hypochondriasis
- depression
- hysteria
- psychopathic deviance
- masculinity–feminity
- paranoia
- psychasthenia
- schizophrenia
- hypomania.

Many other scales have subsequently been developed from the same items, e.g. social introversion. There are also three validating scales: lie (L), validity (F) and correction (K).

The point of view in determining the importance of a trait in this case is that of the clinical worker who wishes to assay those traits that are commonly characteristic of psychological abnormality.

Research with the MMPI has generally taken three forms (Freeman 1976):

1. descriptive studies in which the MMPI performance of the average pain patient (including sex-related differences) is related and analysed
2. diagnostic studies using the MMPI to distinguish between patients whose pain is believed to be functional in nature and those whose pain is clearly organic in aetiology
3. outcome studies using MMPI performance to predict success in the treatment of chronic pain.

The scales were developed by contrasting the normal groups with carefully studied clinical cases. The first three scales, depression (D), hypochondriasis (HS) and hysteria (HY) are the most specifically helpful in relating to medical problems (McCreary et al 1980), and can produce various meaningful patterns and configurations when charted. These have been reviewed in a previous chapter.

There is considerable literature on the use of the MMPI for low back pain patients. Some authors are in favour of its use and others do not support its use (Main et al 1991). However, the reliability and validity of the MMPI has been determined and the major criticism relates to the length of the test. It consists of 566 items and takes over 1 hour to complete. It should also be administered under the supervision of a clinical psychologist and as such is not suitable for routine use in an outpatients' department. In an outpatients' department, use of some of the shorter tests is recommended.

Main et al (1991) identified specific problems with the MMPI, such as obtaining satisfactory completion of the test. This may be a feature of the length of the test or the nature of the items. Specific low back scales or numerous short forms (using all the scales) have sometimes been used as an alternative for the whole test. Although this may be useful in determining certain characteristics such as depression, hypochondriasis and hysteria (Adams et al 1994), some authors have argued that the scales cannot be interpreted in isolation and it is only the complete MMPI profile that is meaningful, and the relationship of the scales to each other.

Main & Waddell (1987) used the Eysenck Personality Inventory and found that simple measures of distress such as heightened somatic awareness and depressive symptomatology (Zung 1965) were more highly associated with patients' level of disability than personality traits. This showed that overconcern about generalized physical complaints and feelings of depression were more related to the resultant disability that the patient suffered than to any particular personality trait. Their results suggest that there may not be a particular type of personality that suffers from chronic pain. Main developed the MSPQ as a response to his critique of the MMPI. The clinical scales of the MMPI can provide useful data with regard to identifying depressive, hypochondriacal or somatizing factors in chronic pain patients, i.e. descriptive or diagnostic uses. However, caution must be expressed in using these results to predict outcome.

Modified Somatic Perception Questionnaire (MSPQ)

This questionnaire was derived by Main (1983) specifically for use with chronic backache patients and is illustrated in Figure 7.3. The simple four-point scale is easy to administer, has high patient compliance and in conjunction with measures of depressive symptomatology and inappropriate signs and symptoms has been shown to be useful in testing back pain patients. The scale was derived from a pilot study of 102 chronic backache patients and its construct validity confirmed on a further study of 200 backache patients. The author integrated sex differences into the final version. The scale was compared with the Zung Depression Inventory and the first three clinical scales of the MMPI. Individual items were compared with clinical symptomatology rated independently by an orthopaedic surgeon. It has been widely advocated by the author. Its simplicity to administer and score makes it useful in an outpatient department to obtain information related to patients' somatic symptoms.

Please describe how you have felt during the PAST WEEK by making a check mark (√) in the appropriate box. Please answer all the questions. Do not think too long before answering. These questions are merely to assess other symptoms you may have in addition to your pain and incapacity. Some of the questions may appear inappropriate but we would like you to answer them anyway.

	Not at all	A little/ slightly	A great deal/quite a bit	Extremely/ could not have been worse
1. Heart rate increasing				
2. Feeling hot all over				
3. Sweating all over				
4. Sweating in a particular part of the body				
5. Pulse in neck				
6. Pounding in head				
7. Dizziness				
8. Blurring of vision				
9. Feeling faint				
10. Everything appearing faint				
11. Nausea				
12. Butterflies in stomach				
13. Pain or ache in stomach				
14. Stomach churning				
15. Desire to pass water				
16. Mouth becoming dry				
17. Difficulty swallowing				
18. Muscles in neck aching				
19. Muscles twitching or jumping				
20. Legs feel weak				
21. Tense feeling across forehead				
22. Tense feeling in jaw muscles				

Figure 7.3 Modified Somatic Perception Questionnaire.

Depression inventories

The Beck Depression Inventory (BDI) is a simple, self-administered test for depression. It consists of 21 items with a cumulative scoring system focusing on such manifestations of depression as sleep disturbance, sexual dysfunction, weight change and mood disturbance.

When the test is used in conjunction with a psychosocial interview, the scores may provide information about the patient's psychological state and approach to pain. High scores may suggest the need for psychiatric or psychological referral. Patients who have high scores on the BDI are often very fragile psychologically. Those with a high BDI score, but very low functional impairment are generally very dependent and feel overwhelmed by all stressors (Capra et al 1985)

The BDI can be repeated at subsequent visits, to chart progression of the patients depressive symptoms and the effects of treatment programmes. The Modified Zung Depression Inventory is recommended by Main & Waddell (1987) for use with the MSPQ to detect depressive symptoms. This 23 item test is easily scored and is illustrated in Figure 7.4.

Illness Behaviour Questionnaire (IBQ)

The concept of illness behaviour was developed by Mechanic (1962). Pilowsky & Spence (1975a), as a furtherance of this, developed the concept of abnormal illness behaviour as a unifying label for all cognitive, affective and behavioural disturbances associated with chronic pain. In order to develop a measure of this construct, the authors administered a 55-item questionnaire to 100 patients with chronic pain of diverse aetiologies. A factor analysis of the patients' responses produced seven independent dimensions:

1. general hypochondriasis
2. conviction of disease
3. psychological versus somatic focus of disease
4. affective inhibition
5. affective disturbance
6. denial of life problems unrelated to pain
7. irritability.

The patients' scores on these derived factor scales were then entered in a clustering procedure that produced three relatively normal patterns of scores and three patterns indicative of abnormal illness behaviour.

There were many psychometric weaknesses associated with the development of the IBQ, including the lack of reliability data and the use of inappropriate factor-analytic procedures (Bradley et al 1993). Although a series of studies has demonstrated that patients with various chronic

Please indicate for each of these questions which answer best describes how you have been feeling recently.

	Rarely or none of the time (less than 1 day per week)	Some or little of the time (1–2 days per week)	A moderate amount of the time (3–4 days per week)	Most of the time (5–7 days per week)
1. I feel downhearted and sad	0	1	2	3
2. Morning is when I feel best	3	2	1	0
3. I have crying spells or feel like it	0	1	2	3
4. I have trouble getting to sleep at night	0	1	2	3
5. I feel that nobody cares	0	1	2	3
6. I eat as much as I used to	3	2	1	0
7. I still enjoy sex	3	2	1	0
8. I notice I am losing weight	0	1	2	3
9. I have trouble with constipation	0	1	2	3
10. My heart beats faster than usual	0	1	2	3
11. I get tired for no reason	0	1	2	3
12. My mind is as clear as it used to be	3	2	1	0
13. I tend to wake up too early	0	1	2	3
14. I find it easy to do the things I used to	3	2	1	0
15. I am restless and can't keep still	0	1	2	3
16. I am more irritable than usual	0	1	2	3
17. I feel hopeful about the future	3	2	1	0
18. I find it easy to make a decision	3	2	1	0
19. I feel quite guilty	0	1	2	3
20. I feel that I am useful and needed	3	2	1	0
21. My life is pretty full	3	2	1	0
22. I feel that others would be better off if I were dead	0	1	2	3
23. I am still able to enjoy the things I used to	3	2	1	0

Figure 7.4 Depression inventory. (Reproduced with kind permission from Main & Waddell 1984.)

pain syndromes or symptoms without organic pathology produce higher IBQ scores than controls, several recent factor-analytic investigations have raised questions concerning the factor structure and scoring of the IBQ. Another factor-analytic study of the 62-item IBQ produced six independent factors that closely resembled the factors originally derived by Pilowsky & Spence. These were:

1. health worry
2. illness disruption
3. affective inhibition
4. affective disturbance
5. denial of life problems
6. irritability.

It was also found that each of the factor scales was correlated significantly with the EPI Neuroticism Scale. Thus, although the IBQ might be able to discriminate chronic pain patients from normal controls, the instrument might measure primarily anxiety or other neurotic features rather than patterns of abnormal illness behaviour.

Back Pain Classification Scale and SCL-90R

As previously discussed, the MMPI is a comparatively old test and has received much criticism (Main 1992). However, many of the newer scales such as the Back Pain Classification Scale (BPCS) and the Symptoms Checklist 90 (Revised) (SCL-90R) have been validated against the MMPI, and correlations have been found by Kinney et al (1991) between corresponding MMPI and SCL-90R scales. However, analysis of the inter-scale correlations of the SCL-90R indicated that it may be a single factor instrument that assesses general psychological distress. Kinney et al (1991) suggested that the SCL-90R may be used as a screening device for psychological distress in chronic low back pain patients, but if more detailed information about the patients' psychological condition is required, the MMPI will be a more useful instrument.

Coping Strategies Questionnaire

Chronic low back pain patients' responses to the Coping Strategies Questionnaire (CSQ) produced three related underlying dimensions:

1. cognitive coping and suppression (e.g. reinterpreting pain sensations)
2. helplessness (e.g. catastrophizing)
3. diverting attention and praying (e.g. praying or hoping).

It was also found that patients with high scores on the cognitive coping and suppression or the diverting attention and praying factor tended to show high levels of functional impairment. Those who produced high helplessness scores tended to display high levels of anxiety and depression.

The Distress and Risk Assessment Method (DRAM)

The Distress and Risk Assessment Method (Main et al 1992) is derived from a simple set of scales validated for use with patients with low back pain. It offers a simple classification of patients into those showing no psychological distress, those at risk of developing major psychological overlay and those clearly distressed. Four patient types can be identified on the basis of scores on two short questionnaires. These are:

1. normal (N)
2. at risk (R)
3. distressed: depressive (DD)
4. distressed: somatic (DS).

Fear Avoidance Beliefs Questionnaire

The central construct of the fear avoidance model is fear of pain. This questionnaire (Fig. 7.5) assesses the tendency to avoid any activity that results or has the potential to result in pain, and therefore avoid exercise or any other functional activity. There are two types of pain avoider (Rose et al 1995):

1. *Adaptive pain avoider*. This type of patient confronts the pain and views LBP as a temporary condition which is inconvenient as the patient is motivated to work and engage in social and leisure activities. Such individuals are prepared to confront their pain as the organic condition resolves in order to continue with their daily activities. Thus they tend to experience a reduction in fear as time progresses.

2. *Non-adaptive pain avoider*. In contrast to the adaptive avoider, the non-adaptive avoider will avoid doing anything to exacerbate pain, and will sacrifice social and work commitments and often avoid physical activity completely. Such avoidance in turn leads to further dysfunction and consequent increase in pain and depression as the person becomes further incapacitated.

Lethem et al (1983) suggest that the tendency to avoid pain is determined by several psychological and social factors such as motivation to work, context of injury, family history of invalidity, personality and previous history of pain.

The validity of the fear avoidance model in terms of explaining chronic LBP has been demonstrated by authors such as Lethem et al (1983) and Rose et al (1992) and is useful in assessing the beliefs of patients who are participating in a programme that will involve physical activity.

Here are some of the things which other patients have told us about their pain. For each statement please circle any number from 0 to 6 to say how much physical activities, such as, bending, lifting, walking or driving, affect or would affect **your** back pain.

		Completely disagree		Unsure			Completely agree	
1.	My pain was caused by physical activity	0	1	2	3	4	5	6
2.	Physical activity makes my pain worse	0	1	2	3	4	5	6
3.	Physical activity might harm my back	0	1	2	3	4	5	6
4.	I should not do physical activities which (might) make my pain worse	0	1	2	3	4	5	6
5.	I cannot do physical activities which (might) make my pain worse	0	1	2	3	4	5	6

The following statements are about how your normal work affects or would affect your back pain.

		Completely disagree		Unsure			Completely agree	
6.	My pain was caused by my work or by an accident at work	0	1	2	3	4	5	6
7.	My work aggravated my pain	0	1	2	3	4	5	6
8.	I have a claim for compensation for my pain	0	1	2	3	4	5	6
9.	My work is too heavy for me	0	1	2	3	4	5	6
10.	My work makes or would make my pain worse	0	1	2	3	4	5	6
11.	My work might harm my back	0	1	2	3	4	5	6
12.	I should not do my normal work with my present pain	0	1	2	3	4	5	6
13.	I cannot do my normal work with my present pain	0	1	2	3	4	5	6
14.	I cannot do my normal work till my pain is treated	0	1	2	3	4	5	6
15.	I do not think that I will be back to my normal work within 3 months	0	1	2	3	4	5	6
16.	I do not think that I will ever be able to go back to work	0	1	2	3	4	5	6

Scoring:
Scale 1: fear avoidance beliefs about work-items 6, 7, 9, 10, 11, 12, 15
Scale 2: fear avoidance beliefs about physical activity-items 2, 3, 4, 5

Figure 7.5   Fear avoidance beliefs questionnaire.

Other tests used in the psychological assessment of pain

Other tests which may be useful in the psychological assessment of pain are measures of anxiety, self-esteem and behavioural health: the State–Trait anxiety Inventory (STAI), Millon Behavioral Health Inventory and the Coopersmith Self-Esteem Inventory.

State–Trait Anxiety Inventory

The State–Trait Anxiety Inventory comprises two separate anxiety scales, each of which takes approximately 2–5 minutes to complete. One scale measures 'state' anxiety, or how one feels at that moment. The other scale measures 'trait' anxiety or how one generally feels.

Because it is easy and quick to administer and score, this test can be used to chart therapeutic progress as well as to assess current status. Advantages of the STAI include wide use, ease of administration and scoring and proven validity and reliability.

Millon Behavioral Health Inventory

This is a 150-question true/false test based on 20 clinical scales that reflect medically related concerns such as compliance with treatment regiments and reaction to treatment personnel. It was devised as an alternative to the MMPI for use with a clinical population.

It is much shorter than the MMPI and therefore does not take as long to complete. It also includes questions related to medical care which patients find less intimidating than questions related to their personality characteristics.

This test is comparatively new and to date lacks substantial evidence to document its reliability.

Coopersmith Self-Esteem Inventory

It has been suggested that low self-esteem may predispose to illness, though the mechanisms involved are unclear. In addition, poor financial status or loss of work as a result of back pain may also result in reduced self-esteem. Depressed patients often have a low self-esteem and participating in a rehabilitation programme may improve mood and confidence.

The Coopersmith Inventory measures respondents' evaluation of their competence, success and worth by rating statements like 'I give in very easily' and 'I have a low opinion of myself'. These are scored on a true/false basis.

This well-documented inventory is quick to administer, taking 2–5 minutes, and quantifies a person's sense of worth and mastery. These attitudes are important to the experience of pain as discussed in the chapter on psychosocial factors affecting pain (Ch. 5). This inventory can be useful for charting progress in this area.

Summary of psychological tests used in assessment of low back pain

A number of psychological tests have been found to be useful in the assessment of LBP. Some are more useful in the early stages of back pain when the clinician is seeking a diagnosis; more detailed or specific inventories may be considered at a later stage if a strong psychological overlay is suspected and the patient is not responding to physical treatment intervention.

Somatic symptoms and depression are helpful to consider at the first assessment and the MSPQ and BDI may be helpful at this stage. At later stages, other inventories may be more useful, depending on what the clinician wishes to investigate.

ASSESSMENT OF PHYSICAL IMPAIRMENT

Physical examination must always be preceded by a medical history. It is also important to consider that there may be patterns of illness behaviour and psychological influences that may affect the physical examination, and the symptoms and signs of physical disease and abnormal illness behaviour should be compared in chronic low back pain patients.

In assessing physical impairment the following tests should be performed.:

1. observation
2. measurement of spinal mobility
3. straight leg raise (SLR)
4. nerve compression signs
5. dermatomes
6. myotomes
7. tenderness/palpation
8. non-organic signs and behavioural responses to examination.

For a fuller description of lumbar examination, the reader is referred to Grieve (1991).

Observation

This plays an important role in the assessment of pain. The patients' gait should be observed and also how freely they move. It is often possible to recognize exaggerated movements and behaviours at this early stage. It should also be noticed whether the patient adopts a depressed posture and facial expression. Ease of undressing also indicates loss of movement and functional ability. When undressed, it is possible to observe deformities, scarring, whether scoliosis or kyphosis is present and whether the lumbar lordosis is reduced or accentuated.

Spinal motion

Spinal motion is important in terms of symmetry and rhythm rather than its absolute values. This is because there is considerable variation in spinal mobility in the normal population and difficulty with obtaining standard-ization and consequent reliability of measurement (Dillard et al 1991, Gill et al 1988).

Lumbar flexion

The common technique of measuring lumbar flexion by seeing how close the fingers can approach the floor and the single goniometer method of how far the pelvis tilts forward are not valid as they fail to separate spinal and hip flexion and may also be influenced by hamstring tightness, nerve root irritation and neuroticism (Borenstein et al 1995). Mayer et al (1984) recommend a double goniometer technique and Waddell (1987) rec-ommends the use of a tape measure. A mark is made on the skin in the midline at the level of the dimples of Venus which approximates L5. A second mark is made 10 cm above and a third mark 5 cm below the initial mark. The patient is then asked to bend forward with the knees straight, reaching both hands as far as possible towards the toes and the increase in the distance between the upper and lower marks is taken as the measure of lumbar flexion. 90% of asymptomatic normal people flex at least 5 cm and this is higher in young adults. Most patients are unaware of the relative movements of the spine and hips as they bend forward and the method includes considerable distraction. It is difficult to falsify this test and it has been found to be almost completely independent of psychological disturbance. This is illustrated in Figure 7.6.

However, lumbar flexion has not been found to be significantly reduced in chronic low back pain patients (Adams 1992) and the movements of lumbar extension and rotation were found to be more relevant in assessing lumbar dysfunction.

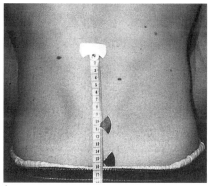 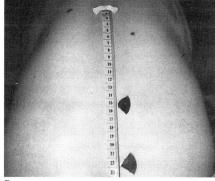

A   B

Figure 7.6   Measurement of lumbar flexion.

Lumbar extension

Lumbar extension is often markedly reduced in chronic biomechanical LBP. This is common because most working postures are in the flexed position, e.g. sitting at a desk or driving. When these postures are prolonged, the soft tissues many become stretched and painful and the patient loses the lumbar lordosis. This then causes unequal loads to be placed upon the spine.

Lumbar extension may be measured using the tape measure method described for lumbar flexion. Alternatively it may be measured using an inclinometer. It is usual to perform these measurements in the standing position.

Lateral flexion

This may be measured by a tape measure using the distance from the tip of the middle finger to the floor when the subject bends to either side or again an inclinometer may be used. Lateral flexion causes ligamentous or muscular stretching and is therefore indicative of a soft tissue dysfunction. However, pain that is increased when the patient laterally flexes to the same side may be related to articular disease or disc protrusion lateral to the nerve root (Borenstein et al 1995).

Lumbar rotation

It is difficult to obtain simple and reliable measures of lumbar rotation. This test is best performed in the sitting position with the arms folded across the chest. The patient then rotates as far as possible to the left and right and the angle is measured. Alternatively, a special goniometer may be used that specifically measures rotation (Mellin 1987). Rotation is frequently limited in LBP patients and often painful. Ths may be due to soft tissue, articular or disc symptoms.

Straight leg raise

The patient should be supine and relaxed with the head on a single pillow. The leg should be raised passively by the examiner who holds the knee straight. The maximum tolerated straight leg raising (to the tolerance of pain) may be estimated more accurately if the angles of elevation are marked on the wall at the side of the examining couch. Restriction of straight leg raising during a formal examination can be easily influenced by psychological factors. Any limitation must be checked in different positions at different times during the examination while the patient is distracted and unaware that SLR is being observed. If, for example, the patient is able to sit upright on the examining couch with the knees straight, SLR is at least 75 degrees. Considerable discrepancies on formal measuring should therefore be noted as possible psychological overlay.

This test should be performed at the same time of day on subsequent visits as it is affected by diurnal variation of the fluid content in the disc.

Nerve compression signs

Standard motor, sensory and reflex deficits occur when a spinal disorder compresses usually a single lumbosacral nerve root. Because of the exact anatomical distribution, they can be easily distinguished from inappropriate whole leg giving way or regional sensory alteration, and even a patient with expert anatomical knowledge would find them almost impossible to falsify consistently.

Dermatomes

The sensory distribution of nerves innervating the lower limb is shown on Figure 7.7. The L1 and L2 dermatomes are a sloping band at inguinal level, around the upper buttock and anterior upper thigh. The L3 dermatome is over the upper buttock and anterior thigh to the inner knee and the L4 dermatome is over the middle buttock, outer lower thigh, anterior calf and dorsum to the great toe over the anterior calf. The L5 and S1 sensory innervation are over the posterior aspect of the lower limb. Differences in sensation bilaterally should be compared to test for any sensory impairment.

Myotomes

Weakness of a muscle group on testing may indicate a disc prolapse at the level where the disc may be impinging on that nerve root. This is common in sciatic-type pains where the lumbar disc prolapses at the L5/S1 level. The L1/L2 nerve root is tested with the patient supine with the hip and knee flexed to 90 degrees. The patient resists trying to straighten the leg. The L3 nerve root innervates the quadriceps muscle and the L4 nerve root innervates the anterior calf muscles. The S1 nerve root may be tested by asking the patient to stand on one leg then raise himself onto the forefoot six times. This is repeated for the other leg. The examiner should stand in front of the patient and lightly hold the patient's hands while this test is performed. Any weakness is indicative of neurological involvement.

Tenderness/palpation

Palpation is performed with the patient lying prone. It should be performed slowly and without hurting the patient unduly. Start by assessing

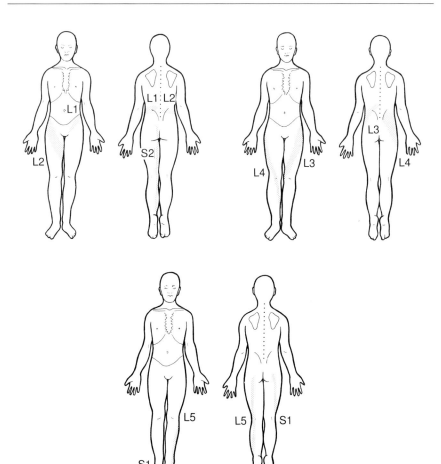

Figure 7.7 Dermatomes.

whether there is superficial tenderness or tenderness to light pinch. If this is present, behavioural symptoms may be suspected (Waddell et al 1980). Superficial palpation should be followed by firm pressure using the thumb tips over the spinous processes and interspinous ligaments 1 cm from the midline T12 to S2. Palpation may thus be used to assess the state of soft tissues, peri- articular tissues and the characteristics of segmental vertebral physiological and accessory movement (Grieve 1991). Deep palpation of the erector spinae may also indicate trigger points within the muscles (Melzack 1981, Travell & Simons 1983). Widespread non-anatomical tenderness is indicative of psychological overlay.

Table 7.1   Comparison of symptoms and signs of physical disease and abnormal illness behaviour in chronic low back pain (reproduced with kind permission from Waddell et al 1984)

	Normal illness behaviour	Inappropriate illness behaviour
Symptoms		
Pain	Localized	Whole leg pain
Numbness	Dermatomal	Whole leg numbness
Weakness	Myotomal	Whole leg giving away
Time pattern	Varies with time	Never free of pain
Response to treatment	Variable benefit	Intolerance of treatment
		Emergency admissions, etc.
Signs		
Tenderness	Localized	Superficial, widespread
		Non-anatomical
Axial loading	No lumbar pain	Lumbar pain
Straight leg raise	Limited on distraction	Improves with distraction
Sensory	Dermatomal	Regional
Motor	Myotomal	Regional, jerky
General response	Appropriate pain	Overreaction

Non-organic signs and behavioural responses to examination

Waddell et al (1980) have identified and standardized a group of behavioural responses to examination which are indicative of non-organic pathology. These include an overreaction to examination, widespread superficial and non-anatomical tenderness on palpation and sensory alterations which are inconsistent with the appropriate dermatomes. These are shown in the Table 7.1. Tests also include the test of axial loading where the examiner applies pressure downwards through the head in standing. This does not stress the lumbar spine and reaction to this is indicative of a behavioural response.

These responses should be regarded as a clinical presentation of psychological distress rather than as malingering.

Electromyographic analysis

Electromyographic analysis has been shown to be helpful in assessing low back pain. Klein et al (1991) found that spinal mobility measurement and isometric trunk strength testing could not be used to identify subjects with and without LBP, though EMG analysis was found to identify correctly subjects with LBP.

Chronic low back pain patients show a higher EMG activity and an altered pattern of contraction indicating hyperactivity in some muscle groups, hypoactivity in others, co-contraction and mass action compared with non-pain subjects. This may indicate muscle asymmetry and imbalance.

In addition, chronic low back pain patients have been found to demonstrate significantly higher motor activity as compared with non-pain subjects (Hoyt & Hunt 1981).

Middaugh & Kee (1987) reported on 23 chronic low back pain patients and found that 61% showed elevated EMG during quiet standing. They noted that 87% showed deviations in rotation and poor recovery from forward flexion when returning to the upright position. The authors concluded that elevated EMG during quiet standing most often represented inappropriate muscle use rather than muscle spasm. This inappropriate use may take the form of either mass action of the low back muscles or avoidance of muscle contraction in the area of pain. Therefore the inappropriate and inefficient use of low back muscles for posture and movement may lead to both overuse and underuse of different muscle groups and the same muscles may show different patterns during different movements. Decreased EMG readings, i.e. hypoactivity of the paraspinal

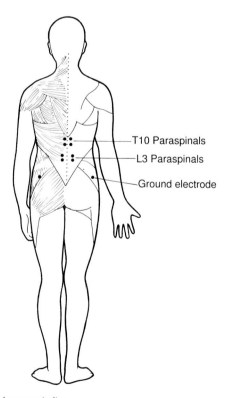

T10 Paraspinals
L3 Paraspinals
Ground electrode

Figure 7.8 Electrode placement sites.

muscles were found in pain patients during flexion and rotation and they showed reduced spinal motion and guarding during these movements.

Motor activity of the paraspinal muscles may be monitored using surface electrodes, and static and dynamic evaluation is required. The positions of the electrodes are as follows (Fig. 7.8):

* *T10 paraspinals.* Parallel to the spine and 3 cm out from the vertebral ridge on a line drawn from below the 12th rib in axillary line to the vertebral ridge. The scanning electrodes are then placed slightly above where the rib cage disappears.
* *L3 paraspinals.* Parallel to the spine and 3 cm out from the vertebral ridge. The iliac crests are first palpated and an imaginary line drawn horizontally across the back towards the spine and the lower electrode placed at this level.

Table 7.2A   Comparison of EMG for pain and non-pain groups at the level of the T10 paraspinals

Posture	Side	Pain $\bar{x}$ (s.e.)	Non-pain $\bar{x}$ (s.e.)
Sit	L	11.4 (1.99)	6.7 (0.99)
	R	13.0 (4.28)	6.93 (1.2)
Stand	L	11.47 (2.9)	5.7 (1.3)
	R	12.81 (2.8)	7.1 (2.0)
S-F	L	12.28 (1.64)	7.73 (1.2)
	R	15.35 (2.56)	7.8 (1.24)
F-S	L	22.36 (2.22)	23.5 (2.9)
	R	27.46 (3.48)	25.1 (3.1)
S-E	L	5.96 (1.22)	4.09 (0.59)
	R	9.84 (2.66)	4.68 (0.98)
E-S	L	9.23 (2.01)	3.64 (0.5)
	R	10.46 (2.4)	3.68 (0.82)
S-LR	L	24.77 (3.25)	32.3 (5.3)
	R	26.9 (3.28)	18.2 (4.5)
LR-S	L	11.9 (2.17)	8.14 (1.0)
	R	18.64 (2.75)	12.1 (2.9)
S-RR	L	22.32 (3.1)	13.59 (2.09)
	R	23.27 (3.7)	36.4 (5.6)
RR-S	L	14.86 (2.4)	9.05 (1.3)
	R	14.73 (2.5)	9.95 (2.3)

Key: E-S = extension to standing; F-S = flexion to standing; LR-S = left rotation to standing; RR-S = right rotation to standing; S-E = standing to extension; S-F = standing to flexion; S-LR = standing to left rotation; S-RR = standing to right rotation.

Table 7.2B   Comparison of EMG for pain and non-pain groups at the level of the L3 paraspinals

Posture	Side	Pain $\bar{x}$ (s.e.)	Non-pain $\bar{x}$ (s.e.)
Sit	L	6.61 (1.2)	4.32 (1.03)
	R	8.84 (3.67)	4.42 (1.07)
Stand	L	13.89 (2.65)	7.96 (1.58)
	R	14.97 (3.83)	7.79 (1.72)
S-F	L	18.6 (2.57)	11.5 (1.59)
	R	21.38 (3.74)	10.8 (1.42)
F-S	L	34.49 (4.64)	27.36 (4.1)
	R	34.9 (4.7)	29.43 (3.4)
S-E	L	7.77 (1.9)	7.14 (2.06)
	R	9.89 (3.88)	7.32 (2.2)
E-S	L	9.24 (1.54)	7.23 (1.87)
	R	12.3 (3.57)	7.09 (2.2)
S-LR	L	22.14 (2.89)	23.68 (3.3)
	R	29.81 (5.7)	30.4 (4.1)
LR-S	L	17.68 (2.88)	13.14 (2.0)
	R	17.41 (2.16)	12.86 (2.0)
S-RR	L	34.45 (3.82)	29.32 (5.3)
	R	31.9 (4.07)	22.5 (4.1)
RR-S	L	20.27 (3.5)	13.05 (2.2)
	R	16.96 (2.3)	11.32 (2.2)

Key: E-S = extension to standing; F-S = flexion to standing; LR-S = left rotation to standing; RR-S = right rotation to standing; S-E = standing to extension; S-F = standing to flexion; S-LR = standing to left rotation; S-RR = standing to right rotation.

Scanning procedures are carried out in both static postures and for the dynamic movement of flexion, extension and rotation. It is important to monitor return from these movements. From these readings it is possible to determine level of motor activity, imbalance between left and right paraspinals and altered patterns of contraction.

EMG studies provide support for clinical diagnosis of the biomechanical aspect of chronic low back pain and this provides the rationale for many forms of conservative treatment intervention. Table 7.2A and B record mean EMG activities for pain and non-pain subjects.

FUNCTIONAL ASSESSMENT

The level of impairment of performance of functional tasks is usually of greater significance than the impairment of specific manoeuvres on clinical examination. It is also of greater importance economically as loss of function affects ability to work. Thus quantification of function is a means of defining disability in physical and ergonomic terms. It may also be used to guide rehabilitation. There are several ways for the clinician to assess function. Some human performance laboratories may carry out a range of functional tests including trunk strength testing, tests of lifting capacity and tests of cardiovascular endurance. For the purposes of this text, only clinical assessment of impairment is considered.

DISABILITY

A number of clinical research groups in the US and Great Britain consider that disability is the best assessment of severity in low back disorders. Disability may be assessed by the extent of restriction of activities of daily living (ADL), and these provide a direct assessment of function which can be correlated with measures of pain and impairment. These activities of daily living generally affected by low back disorders include bending and lifting, sitting, standing, walking, travelling, socializing, sleep, sex and putting on and taking off footwear. The level of disability in these basic activities can then be applied to work, home and leisure activities.

Assessment of disability (Waddell 1987)

1. *Bending and lifting.* Help is required with heavy lifting (i.e. 30–40 lb, a heavy suitcase or a 3- to 4-year-old child).
2. *Sitting.* Sitting in an ordinary chair is generally limited to less than 30 minutes at a time.
3. *Standing.* Standing in one place is generally limited to less than 30 minutes at a time.
4. *Walking.* Walking is generally limited to less than 30 minutes or to 1–2 miles at a time.
5. *Travelling.* Travelling in a car or bus is generally limited to less than 30 minutes at a time.
6. *Social life.* The patient regularly misses or curtails social activities (excluding sports).
7. *Sleep.* Sleep is regularly disturbed by low back pain.
8. *Sex.* Frequency of sexual activity is diminished.
9. *Footwear.* Help is regularly required with footwear.

Simple yes/no answers regarding each of these activities provides a simple, rapid and reliable disability score that is sufficient for clinical purposes.

SELF-REPORTS OF FUNCTIONAL DISABILITY

Sickness Impact Profile (SIP)

The Sickness Impact Profile (SIP) provides a profile of patient functioning in several areas that can provide targets for behavioural intervention. Follick et al (1985) have provided evidence regarding the concurrent validity and sensitivity to change of the SIP scores produced by chronic back pain patients.

Oswestry Disability Questionnaire

This succinct questionnaire was designed to assess limitations of various activities of daily living. It is divided into relevant sections and the patients select the statement which describes their limitations most accurately.

The questionnaire takes about 3–5 minutes to complete and 1 minute to score. Each section is scored on a 0–5 scale with 5 representing the greatest disability. The total possible score is 50 and thus the actual score is doubled and expressed as a percentage.

Fairbank et al (1980) found that the questionnaire is a valid indicator of disability as its score closely reflects the patient's observed disability and symptoms and it has proven reliability and internal consistency.

Interpretation of disability scores (Fairbank et al 1980)

0–20%: minimal disability. This group can cope with most ADL. Usually no treatment is indicated, apart from advice on lifting, posture and fitness.

20–40%: moderate disability. This group experiences more pain and difficulty with sitting, standing and lifting. Travel and social life are more difficult and they may be unable to work. Personal care, sexual activity and sleeping are not grossly affected and the condition can usually be managed by conservative means.

40–60%: severe disability. Pain is the main problem in this group but travel, personal care, social life, sexual activity and sleep are also affected. These patients require detailed investigation.

60–80%: crippled. Pain affects all aspects of these patients' lives. Intervention is required.

80–100%: This group are either bed-ridden with pain or are exaggerating their symptoms. This can be evaluated by detailed examination and the use of tests to distinguish between appropriate and inappropriate illness behaviour.

Other tests of functional disability

Various other measures of functional disability have been developed including the Pain Behaviour Scale, Chronic Illness Problem Inventory and the West Haven–Yale Multidimensional Pain Inventory.

Most of these instruments evaluate variables such as stressful life events, subjective estimates of pain, mood and self-esteem. Although they are multidimensional, their validity has yet to be determined.

Thus it is recommended that both health care providers and investigators use the SIP or Oswestry Disability Questionnaire or other well-validated disability measures such as that of Waddell (1987) to assess functional ability.

ABBREVIATED EXAMINATION

An abbreviated examination for routine clinical use when assessing low back pain patients is given in Figure 7.9.

SUMMARY OF MAIN POINTS.

1. Assessment of the LBP patient should include psychological, physical and functional measures.

2. Psychological tests used in the assessment of back pain commonly include the MMPI, the MSPQ and depression inventories. These test for somatic symptoms and depression and a number of other psychological tests may also be used.

3. Physical assessment of back pain includes measures of ROM, SLR and neurological tests. EMG analysis may also be helpful.

4. A number of tests are available for assessing functional disability such as the Oswestry Disability Questionnaire and the Sickness Impact Profile.

5. A complete assessment is required in order to reach a diagnosis.

Differential diagnosis should lead to differential treatment.

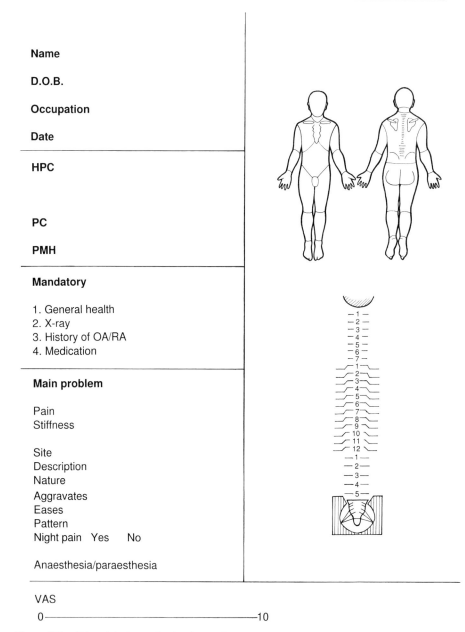

Name

D.O.B.

Occupation

Date

HPC

PC

PMH

Mandatory

1. General health
2. X-ray
3. History of OA/RA
4. Medication

Main problem

Pain
Stiffness

Site
Description
Nature
Aggravates
Eases
Pattern
Night pain   Yes   No

Anaesthesia/paraesthesia

VAS

0————————————————————10

Figure 7.9   Abbreviated examination for routine clinical use. Key: DOB = date of birth; HPC = history of present complaint; L = left; MSPQ = Modified Somatic Perception Questionnaire; OA/RA = osteoarthritis/rheumatoid arthritis: PC = present condition; PMH = past medical history; L = left; R = right; VAS = visual analogue scale.

Psychological Evaluation

Depression Inventory

MSPQ

Other

Observation

General demeanour
Posture/gait
Lordosis
Scoliosis

Objective

Range of movement

Flexion
Extension
Left side flexion
Right side flexion
Left rotation
Right rotation

Other joint involvement

Sacroiliac
Hip
Knee

Leg length

R   L

Neurological

Straight leg raise (SLR)

R   L

Reflexes

	R	L
Knee jerk	R	L
Ankle jerk	R	L

Myotomes

	R	L
L1/2		
L3		
L4		
L5/S1		

Dermatomes

	R	L
L1/2		
L3		
L4		
L5		
S1		

Other Tests

EMG   Analysis

Impression

Muscular
Articular
Discogenic
Psychological overlay

Management

Onward referral
Mobilisation
Electrotherapy
Management programme
Relaxation
Manual therapy

REMARKS:

Figure 7.9 *(cont'd)*

8

Psychophysiological and psychological techniques for the treatment of low back pain

Douglas Taylor   Michael Rose

INTRODUCTION

The previous chapters have shown that chronic pain syndromes involve complex interactions between physiological and psychological factors. Some of the important psychological models of chronic pain and psychosocial factors affecting the pain experience were discussed in Chapters 5 and 6 respectively. This chapter will review and discuss some of the psychophysiological techniques, such as relaxation, autogenic training, biofeedback, and certain esoteric practices, which may be used in the treatment of low back pain, as well as psychological (cognitive) techniques, such as visualization and imagery, hypnosis, and cognitive–behavioural therapies. The importance of the multidisciplinary pain clinic team and back management programmes will also be discussed.

PSYCHOPHYSIOLOGICAL AND BEHAVIOURAL TECHNIQUES

These include:

- progressive relaxation
- autogenic training
- biofeedback.

Current psychophysiological treatments for back pain consist of self-induced relaxation training using progressive relaxation, autogenic training, and biofeedback. Additionally, certain esoteric practices, such as yoga, meditation, tai chi, and chi gong have recently begun to generate interest in the West because of their reported ability to induce a shift from sympathetic to parasympathetic autonomic nervous system dominance, i.e. from a state of tension (physiological arousal) to a state of relaxation.

Progressive relaxation

Progressive relaxation (Jacobson 1938) is an exercise which involves systematically tensing and then relaxing various muscle groups throughout the body, one group at a time, while paying close attention to the feelings associated with both tension and relaxation. This exercise reduces skeletal muscle tension while sensitizing the patient to the subtle differences in muscle tone which denote a tense or relaxed state as they appear in everyday situations, enabling release of tension where it is noted (Bernstein & Borkovek 1973, Bernstein & Given 1984, McGuigan 1984, Wolpe 1973). Progressive relaxation has been reported to be effective in inducing relaxation (Borkovek et al 1978, Danton et al 1984, Davidson et al 1979, Jacobson 1970), but there have been methodological problems in assessing its therapeutic effectiveness. Reviews of the literature have shown an almost universal reliance on subjective self-assessments of relaxation as the principal index of therapeutic outcome (Hillenberg & Collins 1982, Luiselli et al 1979), despite evidence demonstrating a lack of correlation between self-report measures and objective indices of relaxation (Alexander 1975, LeBoeuf 1980, Shedivy & Kleinman 1977, Taylor & Lee 1991). Further, in studies where objective measures have been used as dependent variables (i.e. Burish et al 1984, Carey & Burish 1987, Lyles et al 1982), progressive relaxation was used in conjunction with other techniques, rendering examination of its differential effects impossible.

Despite a lack of scientific evidence of therapeutic efficacy, this technique is widely used by practitioners and has had considerable anecdotal success.

Treatment protocol

A treatment protocol for progressive relaxation may take the following form.

First the progressive relaxation exercise is described to the patient as above, indicating that the exercise is physical training, and, as with any other form of physical training, regular (daily) practice is essential. The practitioner may then explain to the patient that the exercise promotes relaxation because, when a muscle is tensed, upon release of the tension the muscle will return to a resting tone which is lower than the initial resting tone (Jacobson 1970).

It should also be explained to the patient that an habitual state of tension may exacerbate musculoskeletal pain and that regular practice of the relaxation exercise can change the habit of being tense to being relaxed more of the time, which will reduce musculoskeletal pain resulting from ischaemia.

Two important components can be added to the relaxation exercise to increase its effectiveness: one is correct breathing technique and the other is cued relaxation.

Correct breathing technique, which is breathing with the diaphragm and not with the upper chest, is important for effective relaxation. Correct breathing is accomplished through lowering and raising the diaphragm, drawing air into the lungs and then expelling air from the lungs. On inhalation, the abdomen is relaxed and distended which pulls the diaphragm down and draws air into the lungs. Exhalation is accomplished by pulling the abdomen inward by tensing the abdominal muscles, which pushes the diaphragm upwards, expelling air from the lungs.

Cued relaxation involves repeatedly pairing a cue word, such as 'relax' with the tension release part of the exercise so that the body becomes classically conditioned to release tension when the patient thinks or speaks the cue word.

Therefore the patient may be told that the relaxation exercise is helpful for back pain in three important ways:

1. It reduces existing muscular tension throughout the body, relieving pain through muscular relaxation.

2. It promotes the maintenance of relaxation as the habitual body state, facilitating the healing process when structural or tissue damage underlies the pain.

3. It classically conditions the body to release tension with the cue word. The cue word should be repeated throughout the day to increase the time spent in relaxation, as well as to provide a means by which to elicit relaxation in situations that the person perceives to be stressful but where it may not be able to perform the relaxation exercise due to space or time constraints such as when in the office or driving.

Since the relaxation exercise involves systematically contracting and then relaxing different muscle groups throughout the body, one at a time, the patient should be instructed as to how to accomplish the contraction/ relaxation cycle for each muscle group. It is first explained to the patient that, while sitting or lying down, the muscles of a particular group are contracted hard enough to produce mild discomfort, but not pain, while the patient inhales deeply. The contraction is maintained for a count of 3 to 5 and the patient refrains from exhaling during this time. Then both the tension and breath are released simultaneously as the patient thinks or says the cue word. The patient should at all times be paying close attention to the difference in sensation between tension and relaxation, so that he or she can learn to discriminate between each state and favour the state of relaxation.

The sequence may be explained in the following manner, with the addition of correct breathing technique and cued relaxation conditioning.

First, take a deep diaphragmatic breath as you tense both forearms by bending the hands back at the wrists (as if you are pushing something) as far as they will go until tension is experienced in your forearms, but not so it is painful. As you hold the tension, suspend your breath between breathing in and breathing out. Don't hold your breath, just don't breathe out yet. Hold the tension ... hold it ... now breathe out and release the tension, all at once and completely, so that your forearms are completely relaxed. As you breathe out and release the tension say the word 'relax' to yourself. You will repeat this word upon tension release so that your body learns to associate the word 'relax' with the release of tension, so that later when you repeat the word to yourself, it will elicit a relaxation response from your body. Also pay close attention to the difference in sensation between tension and relaxation so that your body and mind can learn to tell the difference between the two, so that later when you make the mental command to yourself to relax, your body and mind will be familiar with the desired state.

Next, take a deep breath as you tense your upper arms by tensing both biceps as hard as you can. Hold the tension ... hold it (count of 3 to 5) ... now breathe out and release the tension all at once, saying 'relax' to yourself. Pay close attention to the difference between tension and relaxation in your upper arms.

Now take a deep breath as you raise your shoulders to your ears as high as you can ... hold it ... really feel the tension ... hold it ... now breathe out and release the tension all at once saying 'relax' to yourself as you let your shoulders fall back to their original position. Really feel the change from tension to relaxation. Now take a deep breath as you purse your lips; press them together as hard as you can, as if you are preventing someone from putting food in your mouth, and hold it ... hold it ... now breathe out and release the tension, saying 'relax' to yourself. Notice the feeling in the muscles around your mouth. Notice the difference between tension and relaxation.

Next, take a deep breath as you squint your eyes as if you are looking directly into the sun and hold it ... hold it ... now breathe out and release the tension saying 'relax' to yourself as you notice the change in sensation in your eyes and cheeks from tension to relaxation.

Now take a deep breath as you raise your eyebrows as high as you can and hold it ... hold it ... now breathe out and release the tension saying 'relax' to yourself and letting your forehead relax completely.

Now take a deep breath as you tense your chest muscles by pressing the palms of your hands together in front of you as hard as you can and hold it ... really feel the tension ... hold it ... now breathe out and release the tension, saying 'relax' to yourself as you release the tension. Notice the change in feeling in your chest from tension to relaxation

Next, take a deep breath and tighten your stomach muscles as much as you can, as if you are preparing to be punched in the stomach and hold it ... hold it ... now breathe out and release the tension saying 'relax' to yourself. Really pay attention to the change in sensation in your stomach from tension to relaxation.

Now tense your thighs as hard as you can and breathe in ... hold it ... really feel the tension ... hold it ... now breathe out and release the tension saying 'relax' as you release the tension. Notice the change in sensation in your thighs from tension to relaxation.

Now, starting with your feet flat on the floor, lift only your heels off the floor as high as you can while your toes stay on the floor and breathe in . . . hold it . . . hold it . . . now breathe out and release the tension saying 'relax' to yourself. Really feel the difference between tension and relaxation.

Now breathe in and lift your toes only off the floor while your heels remain on the floor and hold it . . . hold it . . . now breathe out and release the tension saying . . . 'relax' to yourself as you release the tension. Notice the change in sensation in your calves from tension to relaxation. Notice how the sharp uncomfortable feeling of tension is replaced by the heavy warm feeling of relaxation.

At this point the relaxation can be deepened by going back through the sequence of muscle groups in the opposite direction, slowly, naming each muscle group as the patient is instructed to relax and let go of that muscle group. For example:

Now let go of your feet . . . really let go. Let go of your calves . . . let go of your thighs . . . really let go. Let go of your chest . . . let go of your shoulders . . . let go of your neck . . . let go of your jaw and mouth . . . let go of your eyes . . . your forehead really let go. Let go of your right arm . . . let go of your left arm . . . really let go. Now you are completely relaxed. Whenever you say or think the word 'relax' to yourself, your body will become as relaxed as it is right now at this moment . . . completely relaxed, completely tension-free.

This completes the progressive relaxation exercise. The patient should be taught the exercise during consultations and then provided with audio-taped instructions (the therapist may simply record a training session) for daily home practice, until the patient is able to complete the exercise from memory.

Autogenic training

Autogenic training (Schultz & Luthe 1969) is a system of psychosomatic self-regulation designed to support the central mechanisms responsible for homeostatic processes. This system is based on regular practice of short periods of passive concentration on self-generated psycho-physiologic stimuli, and is designed to facilitate a shift toward relaxation in different somatic systems such as the neuromuscular and vascular systems. The stimuli are phrases such as 'my arms are heavy', 'my legs are heavy', 'my arms are warm', 'my legs are warm', 'my heartbeat is calm and regular', 'my solar plexus is warm', 'my forehead is cool'. Based on psychophysiological studies, Luthe (1969) and Narita et al (1987) hypo-thesize that the therapeutic benefit of autogenic training derives from a self-induced modification of cortico-diencephalic interrelations which enables natural forces to regain their otherwise restricted capacity for homeostatic normalization. This implies that the entire neurohumoral axis (reticular system, neocortex, limbic system, pituitary, adrenals) is directly involved, and that the therapeutic mechanism is not restricted to either physiological or cognitive functions. While thorough research has not been completed on its mechanism, a listing of the disorders that can benefit from autogenic training can be found in Volume II of Luthe (1969).

During the first training session, the autogenic training protocol should be explained to the patient. This involves giving the patient some phrases to repeat inwardly, which help to achieve a state of relaxation and which train the body to maintain a relaxed state all of the time. Such phrases as 'my arms are heavy', 'my legs are heavy', 'my arms are warm', 'my legs are warm' will cause the arms and legs and the rest of the body to relax.

The reason for using the term 'heavy' is because when a muscle is relaxed, it feels heavy; so if the muscles are told that they feel heavy and patients really allow themselves to let go and feel heaviness in a particular muscle group, that muscle group will relax and feel heavy. The more the muscle is told it is heavy, the more that muscle will become relaxed and feel heavy, reinforcing the intention to make the muscle feel heavy, resulting in deeper relaxation in that muscle. In this way it is possible to achieve relaxation in all the skeletal muscles and alleviate ischaemic pain due to prolonged musculoskeletal activity.

The reason the term 'warm' is used is as follows. The peripheral nervous system has two branches, the sympathetic and parasympathetic. The sympathetic nervous system governs arousal when in perceived danger—the 'fight or flight response'. The parasympathetic nervous system, on the other hand, governs the state of relaxation and recovery after the danger has passed—the relaxation response. It is not possible to be in both response states at once; the body is either tense or relaxed. When tense, or under sympathetic activation, one of the events is that the surface blood vessels constrict. One reason for this is that in a physically dangerous situation, if wounded, less blood will be lost if the blood vessels are constricted. This is certainly of survival value in a physically dangerous situation; however, a similar reaction occurs in situations of mental or emotional stress. So when a person is stressed, peripheral blood flow is reduced and the individual will feel cold.

When a person is relaxed, the parasympathetic nervous system dominates and the blood vessels, including the peripheral blood vessels, dilate, so that a greater volume of blood can reach areas which may have sustained damage in an encounter. When the peripheral blood vessels are dilated, the body will feel warm. In the same way that saying and imagining that a muscle feels heavy can result in the muscle becoming heavy and relaxed, when people say to themselves that a part of the body feels warm and they imagine that they feel warmth in this area, the blood vessels in that area will expand to accommodate the visualization and more blood will flow to the area, warming it. When they imagine warmth in many different areas of the body, many of the blood vessels will dilate, sending a message to the brain that the parasympathetic nervous system is dominant. The brain will accommodate this message and shift the entire body into parasympathetic dominance, which is relaxation.

It is important that the patient remembers not to try to relax, but simply have the intention to relax, while remaining detached from the result. This is because the effort involved in trying to relax may increase tension. It may also take some time to achieve this voluntary control over the somatic systems.

It is also important that the patient uses visualization of the sensations of 'warmth' and 'heaviness' such as lying in the sun on a warm beach. It is easier to process these mental images rather than to respond to language in producing parasympathetic dominance.

Thus the patient is reminded to 'let go' and just relax without effort. The patient may be sitting or supine during training, whichever is preferred. The patient is instructed in correct breathing techniques (diaphragmatic breathing) as described in the section on progressive relaxation.

Training protocol

First the patient is instructed to repeat the phrase 'my right arm is heavy', silently or aloud, while imagining that the arm actually feels heavy, using appropriate images. This continues for 3–5 minutes and then the same is performed with the left arm with the phrase 'my left arm is heavy'. Next 'both of my arms are heavy' is practised, accompanied by imagining that both arms are heavy. This practice is continued until the patient reports the sensation of heaviness in the arms.

The sequence that was performed with the arms is repeated with the legs, using the phrases 'my right leg is heavy', 'my left leg is heavy', 'both of my legs are heavy'.

Finally the phrase 'my arms and legs are heavy', is practised, with appropriate imagery and visualizations.

The heaviness exercise may take an entire session to learn, so that the second session may be devoted to learning the warmth exercise, in which the patient is instructed to repeat the phrases as in the heaviness exercise, but substituting 'warm' for 'heavy'.

In subsequent training sessions both the heaviness and warmth exercises are practised and more phrases may be added where appropriate such as 'my heartbeat is calm and regular' or whatever other phrases may be appropriate for specific areas such as 'my shoulders are heavy and warm'.

Biofeedback

Biofeedback is a self-regulation training strategy where a patient is attached to physiological monitoring equipment via surface sensors. These sensors relay information about the internal physical environment which was not previously discriminated by the individual to machines which measure and display it auditorily and visually, making the information available for use in learning to create change in a desired direction (e.g. Brown 1977, Basmajian 1983, Budzynski & Stoyva 1984). Biofeedback equipment will indicate, for example, levels of muscular activity, as in electromyography (EMG), levels of perspiration, as in galvanic skin response (GSR), body temperature, blood pressure and heart rate, and other indices of somatic and autonomic activity. Controlled studies demonstrating the effectiveness of biofeedback in training patients to elicit a shift from arousal to relaxation in central and peripheral nervous system response patterns are numerous in the literature (e.g. Daly et al 1983, LaCroix et al 1983, Mathew et al 1980, McGrady et al 1981), while reports which fail to support the efficacy of biofeedback are rare (Schneider 1987). Biofeedback technology has also provided researchers with tools by which to reliably and objectively confirm clinical diagnosis and assess the efficacy of treatment intervention.

Since patients with low back pain are often depressed, angry, and feel helpless, biofeedback can be an effective way to demonstrate objectively to them that it is possible to attain control of skeletal motor activity with practice.

The biofeedback modality most commonly used in the treatment of low back pain is electromyography (EMG). The EMG machine picks up the weak electrical signals generated during muscle activity and displays them auditorily and visually so that the patient can learn to discriminate between normal and abnormal patterns of motor activity. As a small part of the electrical signal migrates from the motor neuron through the surrounding tissue to the surface of the skin, it can be picked up by the EMG electrodes on the skin over the muscle tissue being monitored. The EMG machine therefore receives this weak electrical signal on the surface of the skin, separates it from other extraneous sources of electrical energy and greatly magnifies it, finally converting it into informational feedback modalities which are meaningful to the user.

EMG biofeedback allows for the direct observation of motor activity in a group of muscles. Very small changes in muscular activity are recorded instantaneously by the machine and shown to the user, who can gain control over these changes by observing muscular activity.

The goals of the biofeedback training are:

1. To be able to achieve psychophysiological relaxation without the machine (Turner & Chapman 1982).
2. To learn awareness of the states of muscle activity and relaxation (Keefe & Shapira 1981, Spence 1984).
3. To develop a sense of control and mastery of somatic systems (Schwartz 1987, Wickramasekera 1987).

4. To gain awareness of stressors as well as one's response style to stress.

Biofeedback may be used:

1. To reduce skeletal motor activity which has been shown to be elevated in chronic low back pain patients (Grabel 1973, Nigl & Fischer Willims 1980, Nouwen & Solinger 1979, Peck & Kraft 1977). In this case the patient learns to voluntarily relax the muscles by observing the changes in EMG feedback as the muscles relax. By practising muscular relaxation, using the feedback to indicate and reinforce successful relaxation from week to week, the patient learns how high levels of muscular activity contribute to the pain, and how voluntarily reducing the muscular activity reduces the pain (Bush & Ditto 1985, Ahern & Follick 1988).

2. To retrain abnormal patterns of muscle activity during movement. A number of studies have found abnormal patterns of muscular activity in LBP patients (Donaldson & Donaldson 1990, Headley 1990, Taylor 1990). Patients showed hyperactivity during certain postures and movement and hypoactivity during rotation. Imbalance was found between the right and left paraspinal muscles during flexion and extension and a lack of reciprocal relaxation was found during rotation. These patterns indicate muscular substitution, co-contraction, inhibition and hyperirritability (Middaugh & Kee 1987). These patterns have been found to be successfully corrected using a combination of specific exercises and biofeedback (Donaldson & Donaldson 1990, Adams et al 1993).

Physiological basis for biofeedback

The sensory inputs from biofeedback are visual, auditory, cutaneous and proprioceptive.

The EMG feedback loop begins with reception of the feedback signal in the occipital and temporal cortex. The signal is organized according to previous experience and relayed to the prefrontal cortex for interpretation and response mode determination. From there, signals sent to the premotor cortex and neocerebellum establish new response patterns through suppressive influence on the motor cortex which inhibits excessive arousal: spinal motor neurons activated by the motor cortex are influenced by inhibitory fibres emerging from the basal ganglia and neocerebellum. Electrodes placed over the muscles under observation relay the amplified muscle signal indicating muscle state and the loop is completed (Wolf 1983). Excessive muscular activity may be maintained via neocerebellar somatic memory which has been conditioned to maintain a high resting state due to structural pathology or psychophysiological stress. EMG biofeedback may help to recondition the neocerebellar motor system set-point to a lower resting state through prefrontal cortical influence on the premotor cortex and neocerebellum which gradually replaces previous conditioning.

EMG biofeedback training

For EMG biofeedback training in the case of low back pain, electrodes are usually placed over the lumbosacral paraspinal muscles. The patient is instructed to relax and 'let go' while maintaining awareness of the feedback. Before biofeedback practice is initiated the patient has already been taught some form of self-induced relaxation, such as progressive relaxation or autogenic training, so that the biofeedback experience is not all trial and error. A biofeedback session may comprise 20 minutes of biofeedback-assisted relaxation training followed by 10 minutes of rest and discussion of the experience followed by another 20 minutes of biofeedback training. Biofeedback training can result in improvements in mobility and pain experience in as few as eight sessions or it may go on for months, depending on the severity of the problem and whether there is structural pathology, such as disc herniation, which is contributing to the pain.

Unfortunately, there are no large outcome studies in the literature demonstrating the effectiveness of EMG biofeedback in the treatment of low back pain, although such studies are underway (e.g. Sherman et al 1995), and reviews of the existing literature show equivocal results (Keefe et al 1981, Nouwen et al 1987). Additionally, biofeedback can be difficult because the principal muscles involved in low back pain, the erector spinae, lie beneath portions of the latissimus dorsi, gluteus maximus, and serratus posterior inferior muscles. In fact, studies comparing surface and percutaneous EMG recordings from lumbar paravertebral muscles have shown low correlations between the two (Wolf et al 1989). When using biofeedback , the clinician should be aware of this and understand that low surface EMG levels in this area do not necessarily indicate low motor activity levels. Alternatively, research supports the use of other target muscles which are remote from the area of pain but which may be closer to the surface and thus are easier to monitor with surface electrodes, such as the flexors of the forearm if monitoring generalized arousal (Johnson & Hockersmith 1983).

Case Study 8.1

M is a 43-year-old man who suffered an L4–L5 disc herniation in a fall down a staircase at his job, which resulted in such pain and restricted mobility that he was obliged to resign from his job and take disability leave 1 month after the fall. The disc herniation was diagnosed by magnetic resonance imaging (MRI), and he was advised to seek physical therapy and stay off work for 2 months. 6 months later, after having tried physical therapy at a well-known rehabilitation hospital, as well as hydrotherapy consisting of mild stretching and strengthening exercises performed while partially submerged in water, chiropractic treatment, and acupuncture, his symptoms were unchanged. By the time he sought biofeedback and psychological treatment, about 7 months after the accident, he had become sufficiently depressed from the constant pain and immobility to show significant and abnormal elevation on the depression scale of the Minnesota Multiphasic Personality Inventory (MMPI) and on the Beck Depression Inventory. The muscles in his lower back were in severe spasm, with electromyograph (EMG) levels significantly above normal. He was unable to engage in stressful situations, and interpersonal relationships were suffering. His back condition precluded employment, since he was unable to engage in any physical activity whatsoever, and he could not engage in sedentary activity without hourly rest periods. It seemed that M would be unable to go back to work until the back pain and depression were alleviated. He was started on a therapeutic programme which included biofeedback, with sensors placed over the L1–L5 region, and relaxation training to reduce the muscular spasms in the area of pain, visualization and hypnosis to help him to control the pain psychologically, and cognitive–behavioural therapy to deal with the depression resulting from the constant pain and lack of success in finding relief even though he had consulted acknowledged experts in the field of physical medicine and rehabilitation.

M underwent weekly sessions of EMG biofeedback training and psychotherapy. Over the course of treatment he showed steady improvement in his ability to control (reduce) the muscular tension in his lower back during treatment sessions, which reduced the pain he was experiencing. After 4 months of treatment the beneficial effects of this programme began to show outside of the office, and he was able to voluntarily reduce the pain he was experiencing by about 60% for most of the day. Because he had structural damage and was reluctant to undergo surgery, he was never able to abolish the pain completely. But the improvement he experienced with biofeedback enabled him to work at a job which required no physical exertion, and the feeling of control afforded him through the biofeedback practice, as well as the renewed self-esteem and feelings of efficacy from getting back to productive work caused the depression to lift significantly.

Case Study 8.2

B is a 46-year-old policeman who sustained a fall at work 7 years ago. He was admitted to hospital at the time with shock and bruising and later discharged. He had complained of episodes of low back pain during the 7 years following his fall; however, this most recent episode had been particularly painful. Previous physiotherapy had alleviated his symptoms only temporarily. Radiography showed mild degenerative changes. On examination, he was agitated and suspicious of the hospital environment. He expressed feelings of hopelessness about his condition and resented not being able to carry out his leisure activities. He had limited range of movement, particularly in lumbar extension and rotation. He had no neurological deficit and reported tenderness on palpation particularly over the right lower lumbar region. B worked under considerable pressure and a litigation case was pending. He showed a significant elevation on the depression and hypochondriasis scale of the MMPI.

Case Study 8.2 *(Cont'd)*

On EMG analysis, he was found to exhibit high static skeletal motor activity, imbalance between the left and right paraspinal muscles in flexion and extension and lack of reciprocal relaxation in lumbar rotation.

B was treated with TENS and specific exercises to treat the dysfunction, which he carried out methodically. He also received stress management and cognitive–behavioural therapy in terms of goal setting and cognitive restructuring. After 6 weeks B had improved considerably. He was relaxed and at ease, his ROM was unrestricted and his pain considerably reduced. His EMG results were within normal limits at this stage. He was transferred to another unit at work where he felt more comfortable. He had also returned to his leisure activities which reduced his depressive symptoms considerably.

When he attended 6 months later for a follow-up appointment he complained of pain on lumbar rotation. EMG analysis showed lack of reciprocal relaxation on rotation. B admitted to having discontinued his exercises due to working long shifts. He recommenced his exercises and bought a portable TENS unit to use as he felt it was needed. He reduced his overtime work in order to spend more time with his family. B thus learned to effectively manage his own condition.

Case Study 8.3

P is a 17-year-old shop assistant who complained of non-specific back pain of insidious origin. On examination, her movements were found to be full, though she was rather slow to perform these movements and she had no neurological deficit or muscular weakness. X-ray examinations and blood tests were negative. P had not responded to medication or physiotherapy. On palpation of the thoracic and lumbar region, her responses were dramatic. Her pain pattern was non-anatomical and her disability far exceeded her physical symptoms. EMG analysis was normal. On psychological testing, she exhibited neurotic, hypochondriacal and obsessive compulsive personality traits.

P was referred to a social worker by her GP as she complained of problems with her housing. It later emerged that P was being abused by her step-father, for which she received counselling. Her back pain symptoms resolved when she was moved into alternative accommodation.

Problems with psychophysiological and behavioural interventions

Problems associated with the use of behavioural interventions (i.e. self-executed relaxation) principally involve client motivation and individual patient characteristics which can affect treatment outcome. Since these treatments rely on regular home practice, compliance can become an issue in unmotivated clients (Carrington et al 1980, Carey & Burish 1988, McGuigan 1984, Patel 1984). Also, it has been reported that patients who show moderate to high baseline levels of anxiety are less likely than are patients with low baseline anxiety to benefit from progressive relaxation and biofeedback (Carey & Burish 1985), and Burish et al (1984) reported that patients with an external health locus of control are more likely to profit from relaxation than are patients without such an orientation.

COGNITIVE AND COGNITIVE–BEHAVIOURAL TECHNIQUES

These include:

- cognitive–behavioural therapy
- visualization and imagery
- hypnosis.

Cognitive strategies, such as cognitive–behavioral therapy, visualization and imagery, and hypnosis, are based on the premise that, with chronic stress, certain inappropriate psychological schemas become conditioned and generalized, forming a maladaptive dominant cognitive framework. This framework perpetuates an over-mobilization of the central and peripheral nervous systems, while the adaptive functions such as objectivity, perspective, and reality testing, become ineffective in counteracting the maladaptive cognitive set. The resultant central and peripheral hyperactivity manifests in psychological syndromes and psychosomatic disorders. The aim of cognitive therapy is to reduce nervous system hyperactivity by identifying and deconditioning the cognitions which form the inappropriate psychological schemas while reinforcing the adaptive functions (Beck 1984).

Cognitive–behavioural therapy

The cognitive–behavioural model of chronic pain focuses on how maladaptive or faulty feelings, attitudes, and beliefs influence the perception of pain, so the therapeutic emphasis is on identifying the maladaptive or irrational belief systems which may be exacerbating or maintaining the pain, challenging the validity of these beliefs, and replacing them with more adaptive attitudes and beliefs. To this end the therapist must first understand the patient's beliefs about the origin of the pain, what the patient believes will help and what will not help, and why. This is important since research has repeatedly shown that patients' beliefs about the effectiveness of a treatment will influence the outcome of that treatment. Also the patients' beliefs about their own effectiveness is important and may require attention if the patient is to make an attempt with a particular therapy.

Cognitive–behavioural techniques for managing pain and/or anxiety and depression which may be present include (Cott et al 1990, Rosenthal & Keefe 1983):

- correction
- cognitive restructuring
- problem solving
- attention refocusing (distraction)
- interpersonal skills training
- stress management.

Correction

Correction is appropriate when an incorrect understanding of the factors underlying the pain exists which may itself contribute to the problem, such as in the case where a patient is tense and anxious believing that a herniated disc may result in permanent skeletal damage or require serious surgery. Thus adequate explanation about the anatomy and biomechanics of the back is required.

Cognitive restructuring

Cognitive restructuring assists the patient in bringing about a shift in thought patterns, replacing maladaptive interpretations of events which lead to helplessness, anger, and depression, with positive and adaptive responses, taking responsibility for thoughts, feelings, and actions. An example of how cognitive restructuring can be useful in the treatment of back pain is seen in the case of a patient who suffered a herniated disc from lifting heavy objects at work and had to take leave of absence from work attributable to the pain. Psychophysiological treatments, such as biofeedback, were proving ineffective. It was subsequently determined that his father could not accept his sexual orientation and repeatedly denigrated him and that his feelings of inadequacy about not being able to work, the accusations of malingering from his father, and his guilt concerning his sexual orientation, all contributed to maladaptive self-statements such as, 'I don't deserve to be pain-free' and 'I am being punished for being bad'. Disputation of these beliefs and replacing the negative statements with positive, healing ones like, 'I have every right to be who I am and who I want to be,' 'I want to be who I am and I want to be pain-free,' 'I am a good, loving person, and I deserve to be pain-free' were an effective strategy for getting the patient to allow himself to be pain-free, and to make the best use of the psychophysiological techniques available to him. Once the negative self-statements were changed to positive ones, the patient began to take a more active role in his treatment and the biofeedback-assisted relaxation training began to have an attenuating effect on the pain.

Problem solving

Learning problem-solving skills is essential to recovery from chronic pain— the patient may need help and instruction in selecting and prioritizing a realistic set of goals for rehabilitation. Often patients with chronic pain have poor problem-solving abilities with regard to everyday difficulties, becoming stressed and overwhelmed by such difficulties. This may result from negative attitudes and low self-esteem. Style of problem solving may need attention as well, as in the case of a patient who was very impatient and rigid in his thinking, so that if a treatment, such as physiotherapy or acupuncture, was not producing relief after a few sessions, he would abandon it as ineffective and try something new. This attitude was obviously preventing him from finding relief, so he learned through discussion that patience and practice and a positive attitude towards the therapy he was undergoing would speed his recovery rather than impede it.

Attention refocusing (distraction)

Several studies have described instances of athletes with severe injuries who have finished a race and then become aware of their injury. Documentaries have reported individuals with severe injuries performing enormously heavy and difficult tasks at the scene of an accident, perhaps to escape from wreckage or to rescue another person who is trapped. This is an example of the principle at work in attention refocusing, or distraction, to reduce the experience of pain. This principle can be used in the clinical setting where refocusing tasks are practised until the patient ceases to habitually attend to every sensation surrounding the pain, as well as to the pain itself, and learns to lessen the pain experience by focusing on something different and more pleasant.

Interpersonal skills training

Patients with chronic pain often have poor interpersonal skills and this leads to them forming poor relationships with others. They often report poor relationships with their partners, and have experienced an unhappy and lonely childhood. These factors may be addressed in psychotherapy and counselling; however, it is important to teach patients to become less focused upon their own condition and to relate to others in a more effective way. Inappropriate pain behaviours are often socially uncomfortable and alienating to others and these should not be reinforced, the therapist focusing on rewarding well behaviours and responding positively to non-pain comments. The patient should be encouraged to engage in hobbies and interests to provide an alternative focus to pain.

Stress management

Stress management is an important part of the pain-reduction program. Chronic activation of the stress response, or 'fight or flight response', can cause somatic nervous system hyperactivity resulting in chronic muscular activity which can exacerbate low back pain. Prolonged stress can also have psychological sequelae, such as chronic anxiety and depression, which can negatively influence the experience of pain.

The stress response begins with the reception of a stimulus by sensory receptors in the peripheral nervous system (PNS) or with an imagined stimulus originating in the neocortex. In the former case, the external stimulus is transmitted by peripheral afferents to the central nervous system (CNS). In the CNS, afferent collaterals diverge to innervate the reticular activating system before reuniting with the main ascending pathways to innervate the neocortex and limbic system (Penfield 1975). If limbic–neocortical analysis of the stimulus results in the perception of danger, a psychophysiological stress response ensues, which includes muscular tension and general overall arousal. In the case of an imagined stressor, the stimulus originates in the neocortex and descends to excite the limbic system, initiating the stress response. The stress response is thus governed by psychological as well as neurologic and neuroendocrinologic systems. Stress-induced activation in any or all of these three systems can exacerbate low back pain by increasing muscular activity.

When a stimulus is interpreted as threatening, sympathetic autonomic efferents from the posterior hypothalamus, which exit the CNS at the thoracic and lumbar regions of the spinal cord, activate sympathetic autonomic end-organ responses via noradrenaline. One of these responses is skeletal muscle tension.

Additionally, sympathetic autonomic efferents stimulate the secretion of adrenaline and noradrenaline by the adrenal medulla. Once in systemic circulation, these catecholamines prepare the body for fight or flight through generalized somatic arousal, including skeletal muscle tension, mimicking the effects of direct sympathetic innervation, but only after a delay of 20–30 seconds, and showing a 10-fold increase in effect duration (Selye 1978).

Recent research also suggests that psychological and psychosocial stressors, such as tasks involving mental conflict or arithmetic (Arnetz & Fjellner 1986), public speaking (Kemmer et al 1986), fear imagery (Lang et al 1980), and visits to the doctor's office (Pickering et al 1988), are capable of eliciting the same psychophysiological stress response as a real-life stressor (Goldstein et al 1982). Further, neutral stimuli can be interpreted as threatening (Lang et al 1980), so it is likely that the greater proportion of episodes in which the stress response is elicited are self-initiated and self-propagated. Stress management helps patients to be aware of the stressors in their life and how the stress affects their pain, to maintain a physiologically relaxed state so no stress response is activated, even in normally stressful situations, and to short-circuit self-initiated and self-propagated stress through cognitive restructuring.

Stress management involves patient education, training in psycho-physiological self-control and life-style modifications.

Patient education. Patient education teaches self-responsibility for well-being, self-awareness and self-assessment of stressors and self-awareness of manifestations of stress.

The first step in patient education is to correct misconceptions about stress and the stress response. Patients should be instructed in the nature of the stress response and the physiological effects of stress such as muscular tension and pain, high blood pressure, ulcers, fatigue, insomnia, skin problems, gastrointestinal problems and others. Patients should also be reminded that they are responsible for the stress in their lives as stress is a result of how the individual reacts to a stressor, rather than a direct result of the stressor itself. Therefore, if it is possible to control the psycho-physiological reaction to stress, then it is possible to control the stress.

A popular misconception about stress is that people think they are aware of when they are stressed. This is rarely true, as individuals are not usually aware that they are under stress until they begin to exhibit clinical symptoms. Research shows a lack of correlation between how individuals describe their physical state and physiological measurements (e.g. LeBoeuf 1980, Taylor & Lee 1991).

Often patients feel that being passive, as when watching television, going to bed or reading, is relaxing. However, the body can also retain tension when in these states, as many pain sufferers find their pain is actually worse on waking.

The patient should be educated about the nature of the stress response, how it is elicited and how excessive or prolonged stress can result in diseased states and pain. Repeated or prolonged stress can result in chronic autonomic nervous system hyperactivity (Cannon 1953), which can lead to hypertension (Reis 1988) and myocardial necrosis (Selye 1978), kidney changes (Folkow et al 1977), resulting in hypertension (Selye 1978) and renal damage (Cromin et al 1978), gastrointestinal difficulties such as ulcers (Selye 1978) and irritable bowel syndrome (Schuster 1983), and vasomotor lability (Sokolov 1963), resulting in migraine headache (Wolff 1963) and disturbances of the peripheral blood supply (Taub & Stroebel 1978). Somatic nervous system hyperactivity from chronic stress (Jacobson 1970) can lead to chronic muscular tension which manifests as tension headache, bruxism., temperomandibular joint (TMJ) syndrome, chronic back pain and other musculoskeletal complaints (Basmajian 1979). Additionally, prolonged stress can have psychological sequelae such as anxiety (Seligman 1968) and can weaken the immune system (Dorian et al 1982) leaving the body vulnerable to infection.

Thus it is possible for a person to exhibit a number of diverse symptoms in response to a stressor, and it should be remembered that pain is also a stressor and these diverse symptoms in addition to the experience of pain can be expected in these patients. Indeed, patients often do report many of these diverse symptoms in addition to their pain. It is important to remember that these symptoms are not merely hypochondriacal symptoms but rather the result of a physiological response to a stressor; in this case the stressor is pain.

Identifying the source of the stressor and avoiding or preparing for these responses is also essential. For example, if a sedentary position is stressing the back musculature and working under pressure also increase muscle tension, it may be appropriate to modify posture or ergonomics and practice deep breathing exercises and relaxation. Training in progressive relaxation and autogenics will help the patient to distinguish between the states of tension and relaxation and to be sensitive to the states of arousal so that steps can be taken to alleviate the condition.

Training in psychophysiological self-control.   Training in psychophysiological self-control is accomplished using the techniques described in this chapter, namely progressive relaxation, autogenic training and biofeedback. Once the patient has learned control over the systems which react inappropriately to stress, then excessive arousal to stressful stimuli can be inhibited voluntarily

Lifestyle modifications.   Lifestyle modifications involve adopting healthy habits, especially in the area of nutrition and physical activity. In terms of nutrition, it is important to eat a variety of foods, maintain ideal weight, eat whole foods and have a low consumption of fats, sugar, alcohol and caffeine.

Physical activity is also important for chronic musculoskeletal back pain patients to maintain aerobic fitness and also spinal mobility and strength. Strenuous activity involving the lower back is not recommended, but mobilizing and stretching exercises are helpful. As it is not always possible to engage in structured physical activity such as cycling or swimming, exercises such as chi gong and t'ai chi described later in this chapter may assist in improving muscle tone, action and strength.

Visualization and imagery

Visualization and imagery refer to the production of mental images which are incompatible with the pain experience. An example of visualization training was applied to an elderly patient who had suffered from osteochondritis (Legg's disease—epiphysial aseptic necrosis of the upper end of the femur which can result in deformation of the leg and hip) since childhood and whose right leg was permanently shorter than his left. The resulting imbalance had caused him low back pain for as long as he could remember. Along with the other techniques discussed in this chapter, this patient was taught to relax and quiet his mind, and then to visualize travelling down a long corridor in his brain until he arrived at a door labelled 'control room'. He would enter the room and scan the banks of computers, which were responsible for the control of all the inner workings of his body, until his eyes came to rest on the computer labelled 'lower back control'. He would approach this computer and select from among all the buttons and dials the dial marked 'pain transmission'. He would reach out with his right hand (attention to detail can make the visualization more real) and turn the pain off, turning the pain transmission dial all the way counterclockwise until it stopped and pointed to 'off', effectively cutting off the pain transmission from the lower back to the brain. He was instructed to use this technique whenever the pain became too severe, and he reported that this technique enabled him to reduce the pain he was feeling by as much as 70%. Of course there are many situations where this technique may be difficult to apply, but if the time and privacy are available it can be quite effective.

The use of imagery to deal with pain is illustrated by the example of a professional violinist who suffered from low back pain during performances for which no structural aetiology could be found. It was determined that performing before an audience was extremely stressful, and the patient would armour herself by unconsciously tensing skeletal muscles, especially the trapezius, which would generalize to lumbar paraspinals. Besides other techniques, such as biofeedback and relaxation training, to make her feel more comfortable in front of an audience, she was taught to imagine that she was not in the theatre, but in her special private spot in a beautiful meadow all alone, with no telephones or other forms of communication so that no one could find her or bother her. It is a beautiful day, with the sun shining down on her, making her feel warm and relaxed. She can smell wild flowers and hear birds singing in the distance. She can watch white, fluffy clouds drift aimlessly by while experiencing the peace of nature and her solitude. As with visualization, of course, effectiveness is increased by adding as much detail to the image as possible to make it real. This visualization seemed to be an effective way for this musician to feel that she was not in a situation where she could be observed and criticized. Of course, the eventual goal was to teach her not to be nervous when playing in front of people, but the imagery helped her in the short term to continue to play concerts while she gained other skills.

Hypnosis

Hypnosis for anaesthesia during surgery began during the first half of the 19th century but was all but abandoned with the advent of chemical agents such as ether and chloroform. Interest in hypnosis for surgical anaesthesia has been rekindled in recent years, however, and a review of the use of hypnosis for pain relief can be found in Orne (1992).

Hypnosis for the treatment of chronic pain usually follows a four-step protocol: relaxation induction, deepening, test suggestions to assess degree of induction, and finally therapeutic suggestions. First, deep relaxation is induced using a behavioural technique, such as progressive relaxation, or by suggestions for deep relaxation alone, such as,

Close your eyes and breath easily and evenly with your abdomen. Breath in clean, refreshing air . . . as you breath out feel the tension leaving your body with your breath . . . do not pay attention to thoughts, but let them come and go like credits on a movie screen. Let go of your thoughts and let go of your body . . . let go of your arms and hands . . . let go of your shoulders and neck . . . let go of all the muscles in your face and scalp . . . let go of the muscles of your chest . . . your stomach . . . your back. Let go of your thighs . . . your calves . . . your feet.

Next, a deepening technique may be used to deepen the hypnotic state, such as, following a sequence of suggestions by the therapist, visualizing oneself descending an escalator and becoming more relaxed with each floor passed so that by the time one reaches the bottom one is completely relaxed. At this point the therapist may wish to test the quality of the hypnotic state using test suggestions for bodily heaviness or numbness. Finally, if the therapist is satisfied with the hypnotic state, therapeutic suggestions may be initiated. In the case of a patient who had herniated a lumbar disc lifting heavy objects at work, suggestions which seemed to be effective in reducing his perception of pain were of the following nature:

When you think the word, 'relax' to yourself, your body will become as relaxed as it is right now, at this moment, and the pain in your back will stop. When you think the word, 'relax' to yourself, your mind will become calm and peaceful, as it is right now, and your body will feel as if it is floating on a cushion of air, weightless, as if you have no body, and you will feel no sensation from your body . . . you will feel only relaxation and peace.

Besides the above 'cued' posthypnotic suggestions, direct suggestions are also effective, such as: 'your back is getting better and better . . . there is no pain anywhere . . . each morning you will wake up feeling fit and healthy . . . when you wake up in the morning there will be no pain at all.'

Problems with the use of hypnosis are that the effects may not last very long and the fact that people show different degrees of hypnotic susceptibility (Orne 1992). Relapse may be dealt with by providing booster sessions, but in those individuals with low hypnotic susceptibility this form of treatment may not prove fruitful.

Difficulties with cognitive interventions

The effectiveness of cognitive interventions in dealing with pain is difficult to assess for the following reasons:

• Cognitive therapy is generally used in combination with other techniques, such as relaxation training, rendering empirical assessment of its differential effects almost impossible.

• Since cognitive schemas vary considerably from individual to individual, comparisons between different reports of empirical findings are inappropriate, and the identification of a homogeneous research population is unlikely.

• Controlled therapeutic outcome studies generally base conclusions on results obtained from a college student volunteer population, resulting in the interpretive problems associated with analogue research (Redd et al 1979).

PSYCHOTHERAPY AND COUNSELLING

The psychotherapeutic approach may involve psychoanalysis, dynamically oriented insight therapy and supportive therapy (Holzman & Turk 1986). In this approach the practitioner may examine the patient's family history in detail, in particular significant emotional events which may contribute to pain. It has been suggested that certain personality types are predisposed to developing chronic pain (Engel 1959) and also those with a family history of abuse and alcoholism (Schneider & Wilson 1985) with subsequent anxiety, depression, low self-esteem and negative attitude.

It is unclear to what extent emotional events may predispose to the development of pain or to what extent they are the psychological sequelae to pain (Polatin et al 1993). Physiologically, patients who exhibit high levels of anxiety, obsessionality and maladjustment also exhibit high levels of skeletal motor activity mediated by reticulothalamocortical mechanisms (Lindsley 1970). Prolonged hyperactivity may lead to ischaemia and pain in the affected area.

Thus the aim of psychotherapy and counselling is to examine the reasons for both physical and emotional pain and underlying anxieties, and to assist patients to develop their self-esteem, confidence and coping skills.

Psychotherapy and counselling can assist in the treatment of back pain in several ways.

• Patients may gain a sense of responsibility for their condition and its treatment through education and insight into sources of stress and the events or situations which may be maintaining or worsening the condition, so that these may be avoided.

• Lifestyle changes may be developed which promote healing and reduce stress, such as changes in diet, time management and avoidance of stressful situations which exacerbate the condition.

• Psychotherapy and counselling may assist in modifying a stress-prone personality to one which is more robust against the effects of stress, which will reduce tension and thus pain. This can be accomplished through helping the patient to change a negative, fearful, hostile and suspicious perception of the environment to one which is more positive and self-supporting, by improving self-concept and developing problem-solving skills.

• The aim of psychotherapy is to develop self-responsibility and independence, and success in this area will help patients to take an active role in the treatment of their condition and reduce resistance to treatment due to secondary gain from the condition, such as the desire to be a victim and to gain attention and sympathy from others by adopting a patient role.

• Psychotherapy and counselling may be necessary to manage psychological sequelae to chronic pain. Patients with chronic pain have often tried many treatments, with little effect. This can lead to feelings of fear, loss of control and shame which can result in a state of learned helplessness and depression. Additionally, feelings of self-worth and self-esteem can suffer in cases where the pain is sufficiently chronic and severe to result in disability, so that the patient is unable to work. For many, the inability to work and the need to rely on society for financial support may be damaging to the sense of independence, creativity and contribution.

Cognitive–behavioural psychotherapy may be the most effective strategy by which to alter patients' negative perceptions, attitudes and beliefs about their condition to positive and coping beliefs and attitudes. Irrational and inappropriate beliefs and interpretations may be changed through correction, cognitive restructuring, attention refocusing, learning problem-solving skills, improving interpersonal skills and stress management. These techniques are discussed on pages 141–146.

ALTERNATIVE TECHNIQUES

Yoga and meditation

Yoga is a system of exercises which include physical movements and postures, breath control practices and meditational techniques, developed thousands of years ago, primarily in India, for the purpose of fostering physical, mental and spiritual health and growth (Patel 1984). The practice of meditation came to the West in the early 1970s in the form of the technique, Transcendental Meditation, which has since been simplified and adapted to the needs and lifestyle of westerners, resulting in various non-cultic forms of the exercise, such as the 'relaxation response' of Benson (1975) and the 'clinically standardized meditation' of Carrington (1984). These techniques involve the practice of physical postures and breath control, along with some form of meditation, which generally takes the form of finding a quiet environment, sitting in a comfortable position with the spine straight, adopting a mental attitude of passive attention, and repeating a sound or word which may or may not have spiritual significance. Studies have shown that the practice of this form of meditation can reduce cardiovascular and neurohumoral responsivity to stress (Benson 1977, Benson et al 1974, Hoffman et al 1982). Other researchers have failed to replicate these findings, and suggest that the beneficial effects of meditation are psychological in nature (Michaels et al 1979, Morrell & Hollandsworth 1986).

T'ai chi and chi gong

T'ai chi and chi gong are exercises which have developed over the past few thousand years in China and other parts of the Orient. These practices involve the performance of slow, deliberate dance-like bodily movements, while maintaining an open, passive mental attitude. T'ai chi and chi gong are designed to alleviate ailments and maintain mental and physical health by unblocking and augmenting the circulation of the vital energy, called 'Chi' (Eisenberg 1985, China Sports 1984, Wile 1985). Millions of Chinese practice these exercises daily, and westerners are now beginning to realize the potential benefits of such practices; however, researchers have yet to show interest in investigating these practices in controlled studies.

THE MULTIDISCIPLINARY PAIN CLINIC

In response to the biomechanical, psychological and psychosocial characteristics of back pain, patients may be referred to a multidisciplinary pain clinic. These are usually staffed by specialist medical practitioners, physiotherapists, psychologists and, sometimes, occupational therapists, nurses and social workers. While each discipline plays an important and unique role, the members of the team work together to address each patient's particular needs and reinforce each other's messages. The medical specialist is usually responsible for physical examination and diagnosis, surgery and medication. Physiotherapists provide education on the anatomy and biomechanics of the spine and are involved in physical rehabilitation. Occupational therapists may provide ergonomic advice.

Psychologists are also an important part of the pain clinic team because they can help the patient to control pain as part of ongoing medical treatment or even as the primary therapy. Psychologists can provide patient education about the psychological issues which are important for the pain patient to understand, as well as providing psychological intervention, such as cognitive–behavioural therapy, hypnosis, and visualization and imagery, and somatic intervention, such as biofeedback and relaxation training. Additionally, many pain patients have psychological problems unrelated to pain which can exacerbate the pain. Psychologists can help patients to deal with these unrelated issues, perhaps attenuating the experience of pain further.

Since many patients present for treatment lacking an understanding of what pain is and what maintains it, an important role for the clinic is to teach patients about pain, because the more patients understand about their condition and the different ways of dealing with the different aspects of their problem the more comfortable and in control they will feel because, at least, someone knows what the problem is and what to do about it. Patients can be taught the difference between acute and chronic pain, possible mechanisms by which treatments can help, i.e. gate control mechanisms, and the relationship between depression and anxiety and pain, and how relief of psychological tension can attenuate physical tension and thus pain and vice versa.

BACK PAIN MANAGEMENT PROGRAMMES

Conservative intervention for mechanical low back pain has traditionally been physiotherapy (Koes et al 1991), back school programmes (Klaber-Moffett et al 1986) and other therapies aimed at reducing pain and increasing physical function. Given the psychological factors involved in chronic LBP, there has recently been a shift towards active coping mechanisms in combined management programmes which incorporate psychological techniques with physical function. These are often based on cognitive–behavioural principles and have reported successes (Harding & C de C Williams 1995, Rose et al 1995). The latter author has developed and coordinates a back management programme at a UK hospital and this is now presented.

The Wirral Back Pain Rehabilitation Programme

Background to and description of the unit

Wirral Hospital Trust, a general acute provider unit serving a population of 350 000, had a growing orthopaedic outpatient waiting list. Analysis of the lists case-mix demonstrated that 30% could be accounted for by mechanical low back pain. It was decided to establish a back pain management programme based upon current trends in back pain management and documented research findings.

Initially, the focus of the initiative were all patients with back pain already on the orthopaedic waiting list. These patients, many of whom had been waiting for 18 months, were transferred to the programme's waiting list. This had the immediate effect of reducing the orthopaedic waiting list by 350 patients. However, patients are now referred directly on to the programme by their GP and a significant number are referred from clinicians within the Trust. The process of entry to the programme was the same for waiting list patients as it is for new referrals.

The unit runs two programmes:

1. A 30-hour (long) programme where patients attend as day patients for 1 full week
2. A 6-hour (short) programme where patients attend for 1 day only.

These programmes were developed at the University of Liverpool and are based upon the studies of Fordyce (1976), Turk et al (1983) and Turk &

Flor (1984) who describe in detail therapeutic interventions designed to address attendant behavioural and psychological issues in chronic pain.

The programme employs a full-time senior physiotherapist, a full-time psychology assistant, a part-time clinical psychologist and a full-time administrative assistant in addition to the programme coordinator. The physiotherapist and psychology assistant are responsible for the group programmes (see below), the clinical psychologist consults individual clients and supervises the psychology assistant, and the programme coordinator is responsible for the assessment of new patients and management of the unit. The administrative assistant acts as personal and clinic secretary and collects data (see below).

On referral of patients, their GPs are asked to complete a structured questionnaire in order to identify serious or surgically correctable pathology. Following the return of these questionnaires, a small number of patients are given appointments to see an orthopaedic surgeon. However, the majority are considered suitable for assessment for entry into the programme.

Patients for assessment are sent appointments and asked to complete a battery of questionnaires which includes measures of disability, somatic anxiety, depression and fear-avoidance beliefs in addition to items concerning severity and location of pain and demographic variables. These measures act as assessment tools and measures of outcome. Variables measured represent the different aspects of back pain experience. Self-reported severity of pain uses a 10-point visual analogue scale anchored with 'no pain' and 'worst pain imaginable.' Disability is assessed using a 24-item instrument developed by Roland & Morris (1983). Psychological distress is measured by two psychometric instruments. These are the Modified Somatic Perception Questionnaire (MSPQ) and the Modified Zung Depression Inventory. The MSPQ has been shown to correlate with measures of anxiety, hypochondriasis, hysteria and depression and has been widely used within the field of back pain research. It has also been shown to have particular utility as a predictor of outcome of an acute episode of back pain. Fear of work and physical activity is measured using the Fear Avoidance Questionnaire (FABQ1 and FABQ2). These instruments were described in Chapter 7.

Patients who attend the assessment clinic are examined and interviewed by the programme coordinator or the senior physiotherapist who have access to the patient questionnaire scores and any hospital notes. The foci of the interview concern the effects that back pain has upon the individual and an exploration of social or psychological factors which may be influencing presentation, and a clinical history. The physical examination is structured and includes testing for 'inappropriate' signs and symptoms such as those described in Chapter 7.

The assessment process enables a decision to be made concerning the appropriate management of patients, and available options include referral to orthopaedic, rheumatological, physiotherapeutic and pain clinics. However, to date, the majority of patients have been managed within the programme.

The long (30-hour) programme

This programme is designed for patients whose back pain disability has become entrenched and who are also experiencing psychological distress (Main et al 1992). Patients are invited to attend in groups of eight and attend for a full week as outpatients with two half-day follow-up appointments at 3 and 6 months. The programme has three components:

- education
- physical rehabilitation
- psychology.

During the week, patients receive education about the function of the spine, the physical, psychological and social dynamics of back pain experience, the theory of pain with an emphasis on the difference between 'hurt' and 'harm' and the general benefits of exercise. Patients are expected to exercise for 1 hour each day but are encouraged to pace themselves according to their individual level of fitness. The exercises consist of mobilizing, circuit and stretching exercises and are designed to improve the mobility of the lower back and to counteract the general physical deconditioning which results from prolonged rest.

The psychology component encourages patients to examine their beliefs about the nature of their pain and aims to challenge unhelpful thoughts about the pain, the self and the future. Patients are also expected to draw up a 3-month goal plan which aims to increase activity level and confidence. All sessions are led by the same two therapists to ensure that the messages being given to patients are completely consistent. In addition, a consultant surgeon or rheumatologist visits the programme for a 1 hour lecture/discussion around issues such as surgery and medication. The main purpose of this visit is to reinforce the therapists' message and add medical credibility to the intervention. The major focus of the long programme is to reduce fear of back pain and facilitate improved psychological and physical function rather than to reduce pain.

The short (6-hour) programme

This is a didactic 'information-giving' programme, the aim of which is to provide patients with the means to avoid future disability. The contents of the programme (which is presented by the same therapist) are based upon the longer intervention but without providing the opportunity for personal goal setting, graded exercise and relaxation. In addition, there are fewer opportunities for discussion and the medical consultants do not attend. Patients are invited to attend for a follow-up appointment 6 months later.

Advice on lifting and handling and posture are not part of the curriculum of intervention as this is considered by the authors to represent a 'medical' biomechanical view of back pain which is not compatible with an approach designed to reduce fear of pain.

Evaluation

Evaluation has been ongoing and has been based upon data obtained from patient questionnaires. These questionnaires are self-administered and are completed by patients at initial assessment, on completion of the long programme and 6 months after attending either programme. The questionnaires provide information on the clinical measures described above, medication usage and some demographic details. Information on 500 patients is now presented.

Initial assessment. Of those invited to attend for assessment, 75 patients (15%) failed to attend. Of those who attended, 140 were considered suitable for the long programme and 148 for the short programme. Of those who were not suitable for either programme, the majority were referred back to their GPs with a smaller proportion being referred for more conventional hospital-based treatment (12% to orthopaedic consultants, 6% to pain clinics and 5% for physiotherapy). The data suggest that those referred to the long programme were a more distressed and disabled group than those considered suitable for the short programme. Those attending the long programme were also more likely to be unemployed (36% as compared with 22%), or claiming sickness benefits (41% as compared with 21%) and to have had a previous hospital-based treatment (60% as compared with 21%) than those attending the short programme.

Long programme. Of those who were invited to attend, 17% failed to attend and 11% failed to complete the programme. Of those who completed the week, 28% failed to attend for their 6-month follow-up appointment. For those on whom a complete data set is available (N = 69), analysis demonstrates a significant reduction on measures of depression (p < 0.01), disability (p < 0.01) and physical activity (p < 0.01), immediately on completion of the programme and at 6-month follow-up. There was also a significant reduction in the use of analgesic and anti-inflammatory medications 6 months after the programme.

Short programme. Of those who were invited to attend the short programme, 22% failed to attend, and of those who completed the programme, 41% failed to attend for 6-month follow-up. For those on whom a complete data set is available (N = 68), analysis demonstrated a significant reduction on measure of disability (p < 0.01), fear of physical activity (p < 0.01) and use of analgesics (p < 0.01) at 6-month follow-up.

Conclusions

The initial audit suggests that the programme is effective in a number of ways.

1. Patients who attend either of the programmes appear to be more active and less frightened, and those attending the long programme, less depressed than prior to attending a programme.
2. Patients at the end of either of the programmes seem to use less medication than prior to the programmes. It may be suggested that these changes reflect a shift away from passive coping strategies such as rest and taking medication to a more active coping style, characterized by exercise and increased functional activity.
3. Subsequently, patients feel less need to consult the medical profession for help with their back pain and therefore reduce pressure on already stretched health resources.

The *Clinical Standards Advisory Group* (*CSAG*) report recommends that every purchaser should have a specific contract for the provision of a back pain rehabilitation service, and its description of a service closely resembles that of the Wirral Hospital. The report also comments, however, that GPs seem reluctant to contract services for patients with low back pain, preferring to concentrate on areas where gains are more directly measurable. There are limitations to the conclusions which can be drawn from this evaluation, which result in the most part from the practical difficulties of conducting a scientific and controlled study in a hospital setting. However, the initial audit of the service shows that the benefits of such a programme both to patients and to the Trust can be demonstrated in measurable ways.

Summary

In this chapter some of the psychophysiological and psychological techniques which may be used in the treatment of low back pain have been reviewed and discussed. Psychophysiological techniques discussed include relaxation training procedures such as progressive relaxation, autogenic training and biofeedback. Certain esoteric practices which have recently begun to receive attention in the literature include health-promoting practices such as yoga and meditation and the oriental healing practices t'ai chi and chi gong are also reviewed. Psychological interventions discussed include cognitive–behavioural techniques such as correction, cognitive restructuring, problem solving, attention refocusing (distraction), interpersonal skills training and stress management. Visualization, imagery and hypnosis are also discussed as psychological interventions for low back pain.

The importance of the multidisciplinary pain clinic team and back management programme is also discussed.

SUMMARY OF MAIN POINTS

1. A number of psychophysiological and psychological techniques may be used in the treatment of low back pain. These include psycho-physiological techniques, cognitive–behavioural techniques, psychotherapy and counselling and alternative techniques.

2. Psychophysiological techniques include progressive relaxation, autogenic training and biofeedback. Progressive relaxation is an exercise which involves systematically tensing and relaxing various muscle groups throughout the body to induce relaxation. The use of cued relaxation and correct (diaphragmatic) breathing increase therapeutic efficacy.

3. Autogenic training is a system of psychosomatic self-regulation and is designed to facilitate a shift towards relaxation in different somatic systems. Certain phrases are repeated and visualization of sensations such as warmth and heaviness in the muscles is used to facilitate a state of parasympathetic dominance, i.e. relaxation.

4. Biofeedback is a self-regulation training strategy where a patient is attached to physiological monitoring equipment via surface electrodes. These electrodes relay information about levels of muscular activity as in EMG, blood pressure, heart rate and other indices of somatic and autonomic activity. Patients can then be taught to alter their responses appropriately and attain control of these activities. Biofeedback technology has also provided researchers with tools by which to reliably and objectively confirm clinical diagnosis and assess outcomes of treatment.

5. Cognitive and cognitive–behavioural techniques include cognitive behavioural therapy, visualization and imagery, and hypnosis. The aim of cognitive therapy is to reduce nervous system hyperactivity by identifying and deconditioning the cognitions which form the inappropriate psychological attitudes, beliefs and behaviours, while reinforcing adaptive ones.

Cognitive–behavioural techniques used in managing pain include correction, cognitive restructuring, problem solving, attention refocusing, interpersonal skills training and stress management.

6. Visualization and imagery refer to the production of mental images which are incompatible with the pain experience. Hypnosis involves relaxation induction, deepening, test suggestion to assess degree of induction and finally therapeutic suggestions.

7. Psychotherapy and counselling may involve psychoanalysis, dynamically oriented insight therapy and supportive therapy. The aim is to examine the reasons for both physical and emotional pain and to assist patients to develop their self-esteem, confidence and coping skills.

8. Alternative techniques. Certain esoteric practices have been reputed to be helpful in assisting relaxation and improving spinal mobility and function. These may include Oriental concepts and meditation.

9. Back management programmes have proved successful in managing chronic low back pain. These programmes incorporate psychological techniques, such as examining patients' cognitions regarding pain, patient education, and physical techniques, such as exercise, to increase physical function and reduce fear of activity.

9

Psychological factors in patient–practitioner interactions

Nicola Adams

INTRODUCTION

In this chapter there will be emphasis on the psychological approach of the practitioner who is carrying out a physical treatment. The psychological implications and outcomes of the practitioner providing patients with a feeling of control and responsibility for their pain and its management will be discussed. There will also be discussion of the importance of the patient–practitioner relationship and the use of interpersonal skills in the reduction of anxiety, fear and uncertainty which all heighten the experience of pain through corticoreticular mechanisms discussed previously.

The use of nonverbal behaviours and of touch, the provision of explanation and reassurance, and the relevance of empathy and rapport to patient compliance and satisfaction, and thus to treatment outcomes, will be discussed. The way in which these skills may be incorporated into clinical practice will be presented.

COMMUNICATION IN THE THERAPEUTIC ENCOUNTER

Communication is an integral part of any professional practice. The potential benefits of improved communication include greater patient satisfaction, better patient cooperation with treatment regimes, reduced anxiety and distress, quicker recovery from surgery and illness and shorter lengths of stay in hospital. These are all clearly worthwhile aims, as better patient cooperation in treatment and shorter hospital stays can also save a great deal of money. Thus, good communication can be justified in terms not only of greater satisfaction and reduced distress but also of cost-effectiveness.

The impact of poor communication extends to its indirect effects. Inadequacies of medical communication may lead to incorrect diagnoses and incorrect or rejected treatment or advice. Dissatisfaction with practitioners who do not seem to care or who will not listen or explain matters is the source of many patient complaints, inquiries or litigation, which are additional costs of poor communication.

In a survey that was conducted in New Zealand in 1989, the four qualities that the public rated most highly in doctors were as follows (Buchanan 1991):

1. listening
2. explaining adequately
3. spending time in the consultation
4. being caring.

Havelock (1991) found that the most common views of dissatisfaction among patients were firstly the feeling of being rushed when with the doctor, secondly the doctor lacking understanding of their condition and thirdly patients' poor comprehension of advice or medication instructions.

Communication is of particular importance in patient–therapist interactions as therapists may spend up to 1 hour in a single consultation with a patient. The outcomes of treatment are frequently dependent on the patients' compliance with home exercises and instructions. Therefore it is important that patients understand the purpose of this advice and how this relates to their condition. In a survey carried out by Adams et al (1994) it was found that greatest patient satisfaction and compliance was achieved when patients felt that they had had adequate explanation from the therapist and understood the purpose of their exercises and instructions. They reported that although not completely cured, they felt better able to cope and, as such, patients were satisfied to be discharged. It is obviously important for the therapist to convey to patients that they may never achieve full function if their condition is chronic or degenerative.

BEHAVIOURS IN MEDICAL COMMUNICATION

In medical communication two types of behaviour are thought to be important. These are instrumental behaviour and affective behaviour (Bensing & Dronkers 1992). They correspond with the two main purposes the doctor has in the medical consultation, which are first information exchange which is necessary for solving the medical problem, and secondly creating a therapeutic relationship which is necessary for managing the psychosocial aspects of health problems and gaining the confidence of the patient (DiMatteo 1979).

Instrumental or task-oriented behaviours are technically based skills used in problem solving which are the basis of the expertness for which the practitioner is consulted. This includes providing information, questioning and directing the patient through the consultation. Giving information is defined as all information statements related to medical condition, therapeutic regimen, lifestyle or feelings.

Affective behaviours are referred to as behaviours with an emotional content. This may include behaviours such as showing agreement with the patient, paraphrasing and reflecting the patient's messages, legitimizing the patient's behaviours and showing partnership with the patient. Showing concern and empathy for the patient is also categorized as an affective behaviour. These behaviours may have a strong nonverbal component.

Engel (1988) stated that the patient has two needs in the medical consultation. The first is the need to know what the matter is, i.e. what causes the pain and how this can be remedied. The second is the need to know that he is accepted by the doctor as a person and is not seen as a malingerer. Therefore it is important for the practitioner not only to diagnose and treat the medical condition but also to legitimize the patient's feelings and make the patient feel understood. This is achieved through effective communication. Research has shown that effective communication improves outcomes of treatment directly and indirectly. If patients understand the purpose of their medical condition they are more likely to comply, and thus the outcomes are likely to be more favourable. If psychosocial aspects are addressed satisfactorily, then patients are more likely to be satisfied with their treatment. The components of effective communication have been identified by Adams et al (1994) to include provision of information and empathy.

Provision of information

The transmission of information about illness and treatment between clinicians and patients may affect the quality of care in several ways. The success of a therapeutic regimen usually depends on the patient's compliance with the instructions that have been given (Francis et al 1969). Studies such as those of Wolfer & Davies (1970) have demonstrated a positive relationship between receipt of information about a treatment procedure and decrease in its undesirable side-effects. Additionally, the ability of patients to contribute to a diagnosis by providing an accurate history depends largely on their understanding of their previous illness. Patient satisfaction with information about their illness and its treatment may increase compliance, and reduce the number of consultations, demands for a second opinion and perhaps malpractice suits (Mathews 1983). Problems in practitioner–patient transactions lie partly in the fact that they do not share medical knowledge and language equally. Thus their goals and interests may not coincide. A major constraint on communication in clinical settings is that, because of the technical and specialized nature of medical knowledge, patients generally lack the means to successfully negotiate their interests, i.e. they may not possess the language to ask for information nor be able to process what they are told in a meaningful way. The reliance of medical personnel on jargonistic language often means that patients have a limited understanding of medical explanations.

Sociolinguistic studies of working-class patients conclude that their ability to understand technical terms prevents them from asking questions (Cartwright 1964, Korsch & Negrete 1972). Similarly, they are viewed as reluctant to give information (Mathews 1983). The latter author suggested that patients do not know what information is expected of them as they are not aware of the structure of the medical interview and the types of information the physician requires in order to make a diagnosis. Goffman (1961) observed that the physician makes an assessment of patients' ability to understand medical explanations, which is based on social class and level of education. Higher social class and educational level apparently create the impression that patients are capable of understanding medical explanations because physicians communicate more with these patients (Pendleton & Bochner 1980). Within the clinical setting, patients appear to receive a variety of contextual clues which inform them that their inquiries are not welcomed by staff, e.g. physicians continue talking without paying attention to the patients' 'input' (Quint 1965). Topics may be shifted to avoid sensitive issues and technical language and euphemisms may be used. Quint (1965) and Roth (1963) observed that nonverbal cues included walking away from patients without giving a response to questions, limiting the time available for a consultation and maintaining a spatial distance, especially from bed-patients, which inhibits conversation.

Korsch et al (1968) and Boreham & Gibson (1978) reported patients' needs for information to include information about the nature and course of their illness and impending treatment plans, the process and after-effects of diagnostic and therapeutic procedures, and hospital routines. Since it is likely that patients receive some information about these interests, the communication gap they perceive must be attributable to factors such as the timing and level of information, the attitudes conveyed by staff and problems in use of language (Mathews 1983). Friedson (1970) observed that physicians control information temporally by withholding information about the possible treatment options and revealing their plan to the patient one stage at a time. Boreham & Gibson (1978) found that physicians gave only a minimal explanation of the diagnosis in 50% of the cases and seldom remarked on the cause or expected course of the illness. In only half the cases was the patient told the names and effects of prescribed drugs. The authors found the majority of patients viewed information about their illness as an important facet of the medical consultation, yet few asked for a diagnosis or the name of a prescribed drug. They observed that doctors' response to patients' questions frequently conveyed to patients that they have implied a lack of confidence in the doctors' judgement.

Therefore it is important for the practitioner to provide an explanation of the nature and course of the illness, using as few technical and jargonistic terms as possible.

Mathews (1983) theorized that the reason why some patients do not seek information may be different orientations to patient care. Some patients concentrate on obtaining attention and sympathy while others see the hospital as a place where tasks must be carried out to effect cure, and these latter patients are more likely to question staff about their condition. The author suggested that patients refrain from asking questions due to their impressions that staff are busy and overworked, fear of negative reactions from staff, perceptions of social distance between themselves and physicians and inability to understand medical jargon. Patients may also withhold information from medical staff. Bain (1976) found that the largest volume of patient communication was to relate symptoms, not sociological factors of how the illness will affect them or their family. Cicourel (1981) suggested that patients relied on cues from the physician about the degree of disclosure which was expected. As patients do not know what information they need to provide in order for the practitioner to make a diagnosis, it is important for the practitioner to be structured in the clinical interview to obtain both medical and psychosocial information.

McIntosh (1974) and Waitzkin & Stoeckle (1972) suggested that patients tend to be dissatisfied with the information they receive from medical personnel. Roth (1963) found that hospitalized patients want information about the probable course of their illness, diagnostic and treatment procedures and the social rules of the hospital. The literature further suggests that much of this information is withheld from patients by formal and informal policies which are largely based on tradition, myth and physician preference.

Empathy

Patients also need to feel understood as people and the practitioner normally communicates this empathy through nonverbal behaviours such as maintaining eye contact, nodding agreement while the patient is speaking, appropriate use of touch and a sympathetic voice tone (Hamilton-Duckett & Kidd 1985). Empathy is also conveyed by providing clear information about the patient's condition and involving the patient in the treatment process (Adams et al 1994).

Nonverbal communication

Strecher (1984) observed that 7% of emotional communication is evinced via verbal behaviour and 22% is transferred by voice tone. However, 55% is evinced by nonverbal behaviours such as eye contact, body positioning, touch, etc. Thus, in the therapeutic encounter the affective aspects of the encounter are conveyed for the most part by nonverbal behaviour.

According to Dickson et al (1989), the functions of nonverbal communication are:

- to replace speech
- to complement the verbal message
- to regulate and control the flow of communication
- to provide feedback
- to help define relationships between people
- to convey emotional states.

Nonverbal communication involves:

- Facial expression, gaze and eye contact indicate interest in the patient and concern for the patient's welfare.
- Spatial behaviour. The practitioner should be seated close to the patient but not so close as to encroach upon personal space. The placing of a desk between patient and practitioner implies distance and may be appropriate on certain occasions.
- Touch is used both for therapeutic purposes such as examination or treatment procedures and to reassure patients by conveying caring and warmth.
- Silence while the patient is talking indicates listening and reflecting upon what the patient has said. Patients often feel that the practitioner has taken time to consider their individual condition and circumstances.
- Appearance. A neat, tidy appearance gives an appearance of professionalism and competence. More importantly, the general demeanor of the practitioner in terms of sympathetic manner and courtesy often contributes to the patient's response to treatment.

CONSULTATION SKILLS

Pendleton et al (1984) recommended that consultation skills should involve:

1. defining the patient's problem, taking consideration of all contributing factors
2. selecting an appropriate action based on these findings
3. involving the patient in the management of the condition by establishing a relationship with the patient that is based on a mutual understanding and responsibility for the problem.

Anecdotal evidence would suggest that therapists may communicate more effectively with patients than doctors because of the nature of their treatment. This may be due to factors such as the length of the consultations, of which the first is likely to be most similar to the medical consultation where the purpose is to determine the nature of the problem, the contributing factors, a plan for treatment and a provisional prognosis, e.g. physiotherapy treatment not only involves examination but the therapist also performs the advocated treatment in subsequent consultations. Patient reports suggest that they often form a closer relationship with their physiotherapist than with any other member of the health care team. This may in part be due to the length and numbers of consultations which necessitates considerable touching and handling of the injured area.

Improving consultation skills

Pendleton et al (1984) recommended a seven-task approach to improving consultation skills.

Task 1.   The purpose of this task is to define the reasons for the patient's attendance, including the nature and history of the problem, the aetiology, the patient's ideas, concerns and expectations, and the effects of the problems.

Task 2.   The purpose of this task is to consider other contributing factors and risk factors.

Task 3.   Choose an appropriate action with each patient for each problem.

Task 4.   Achieve a shared understanding of the problem with the patient.

Task 5.   Involve the patient in the management plan and encourage acceptance of appropriate responsibility.

Task 6.   Use time and resources appropriately both in the consultation and in the long term.

Task 7.   Establish and maintain a relationship with the patient which helps to achieve the other tasks.

Ley et al (1973) found patient recollection of the therapeutic regimen to be greatly improved if the doctor separated it from other statements and stressed the importance of remembering the information. They also recommended that directions be given to the patient at the beginning of the interview.

Ley (1972) advised that the message be clustered into:

1. what is wrong
2. what the treatment will be
3. what the patient must do to help himself
4. what the outcome will be.

COMMUNICATION IN PHYSIOTHERAPY

The physiotherapeutic encounter differs from the medical consultation in a number of ways. First the therapist is usually female, secondly the nature of the physiotherapy treatment involves a considerable amount of touching, thirdly the consultation tends to be much longer and fourthly much of physiotherapy treatment is concerned with patients' active participation in carrying out exercises at home.

Wagstaff (1982) observed that a fundamental problem in physiotherapy is encouraging patients to carry out advice and instructions correctly, especially in the absence of a therapist as when home exercises are prescribed. He suggested that the reasons why patients may not carry out instructions are first that patients may not understand what they have been asked to do and secondly that patients are not motivated to carry out instructions.

Wagstaff recommended clarifying instructions and using gentle persuasion to convince patients that the instructions are not harmful or useless but are actually beneficial and worth carrying out.

Zimbardo et al (1977) recommended that to communicate instructions effectively, the therapist should be credible, i.e. the patient should actually trust or believe the therapist. It is known that rank or status increases credibility. They recommended that therapists should never give the impression that they are incompetent or not really sure of what they are doing. The personal attractiveness of therapists in terms of their general demeanor of friendliness, sympathy and concern was also considered important in communicating instructions effectively. Wagstaff (1982) stated that the more patients were satisfied with those who treated them, the more likely they were to follow advice.

Another feature of communication of instructions to patients is the patients' level of understanding of those instructions. Boyle (1970) found that therapists tended to overestimate patients' knowledge and that their lack of knowledge is inconsistent.

Thus, the therapist could be easily misled into thinking that the patient understands more than he or she actually does. For example Boyle found that 57% of patients could not correctly locate their heart and 80% could not correctly locate their stomach. Ley & Spelman (1967) found that 91% of patients knew of the relationship between smoking and lung cancer, and 73% knew of treatment for cancer; however, 30% of patients thought that lung cancer was not very serious and could easily be cured. Dickson & Maxwell (1987) realized the significance of the interpersonal dimension in physiotherapy practice and the necessity for social skills to enable rapport to be established. This and the maintenance of appropriate relationships and effective communication with patients and significant others has been regarded as being fundamental to the therapeutic process by authors such as Lowe (1970), Wagstaff (1982) and Payton (1983). The physiotherapist is required to use social skills when interviewing (Croft 1980), counselling (Grant 1979) and instructing (Wagstaff 1982). These social skills are in addition to the traditionally recognized cognitive and technical abilities and complement these components of the therapeutic encounter.

The role of touch

Of all the nonverbal components of the therapeutic encounter, touch is clearly one of the most influential behaviours as it carries profound and varied meanings and interpretations. The most obvious purpose of touch in the medical and therapeutic encounter is to medically examine the patient. A second equally important function of touch is reassurance. Montagu (1978) stated that touch is the most basic form of communication in that it is fundamental to human development. Cassileth (1980) and Maguire (1985) observed that the person who is frightened and insecure, such as a patient awaiting an operation or who has been diagnosed as suffering from a terminal or debilitating illness, has a greater need of closer physical contact than the person who is strong and independent. In a comparison of medical students' perceptions and attitudes to touch as a form of communication in medical schools in the Netherlands and in England, marked differences appeared. Female students in both countries were more inclined to appreciate the significance of touch in communication but were less comfortable about the breaking of bad news. The British felt that touch eased communication, especially with very ill patients, significantly more than the Dutch, who saw this as an invasion of personal privacy. This clearly has implications in the patient–practitioner encounter as the practitioner is often of the opposite sex to the patient.

It is argued that there is a symbolic relationship with female practitioners, who handle the patient's injured part when the patient is undressed to expose this injured area to a maternal authority figure. A male physician, who the patient frequently reveres, may be likened to a paternal figure (Adams et al 1994). Because of the psychological aspects of being touched by and undressed in front of an authority figure, i.e. there is no sexual component, many clinicians will report that it is on physically handling the patient that the patient will disclose much personal information which may be a contributing factor to their condition. This would confirm the views of Montagu (1978) who stated that touch was the most basic form of communication.

Professional anecdotal evidence suggests that the greater the amount of physical handling and close physical proximity required (as in the case of neurological patients), the less the amount of affective behaviours employed. Although the physiotherapeutic encounter requires considerable physical handling, the therapist generally only touches for therapeutic reasons. Adams et al (1994) found that the therapist spends little time on social routines and general conversation with the patient in comparison with treatment-oriented conversation. The therapist in this way maintains a professional distance from the patient by using brief greeting and farewell statements at the beginning and end of the consultation. This is in contrast with the social situation where close physical contact implies personal intimacy. These social 'rules' appear to be waived in the case of babies, where the therapist acts as a non-discriminative 'parent' engaging in much physical handling and affection as well as the process of treatment.

COMPLIANCE

Many authors have stressed the importance of patients' compliance with doctors' instructions in the process of treatment. However, it was found in studies such as those of Davis (1966) and Stimson (1974) that there is a high percentage of patients who fail to follow their doctors' instructions. Patient compliance was found to be especially poor in the case of outpatients who were not under the immediate control of medical staff. As physicians' attempts to ensure patient compliance are often insufficient, behavioural researchers such as Heszen-Klemens & Lapinska (1984) have tried to explain the problems of patient compliance from a psychosocial perspective. They found that patients were unable to implement doctors' advice if they were not able to understand or remember it. Golden & Johnston (1970) showed that many patients misunderstood what the doctor said because of their emotional reactions to illness or because of cognitive limitations. It has been demonstrated by Brody (1980), Hulka et al (1976) and Ley & Spelman (1965) that at least 50% of doctors' instructions are not remembered by the patient. Even if a doctor's advice is remembered, it is possible that a patient will not follow it for some other reasons. Davis (1968, 1971) found a number of interaction categories connected with patients' compliance. He found that compliance deteriorated when an exchange of roles was observed between the doctor and the patient. Tension or conflict in socioemotional aspects of the medical condition also negatively influenced patients' compliance. On the other hand, compliance was found to be better when both participants acted according to their roles and when the socioemotional aspects were addressed satisfactorily. Davis also found that the doctor's manner of gathering and giving information also affected patients' compliance. Compliance decreased when doctors requested information from patients and did not disclose information themselves. Conversely, compliance increased when information was imparted from the doctor to the patient.

Heszen-Klemens & Lapinska (1984) suggested that the most important factor for health improvement (evaluated on the basis of patients' complaints) was probably the emotional exchange with the doctor, although the exchange of information between the doctor and the patient was an important factor influencing the results of treatment obtained. Warm, directive behaviour of the doctor towards the patient has been shown to have a positive influence on patients' health status measured by decrease of patients' complaints and improvement of objective medical signs and symptoms. Heszen-Klemens & Lapinska concluded that to cure effectively, the doctor should be an authoritative, powerful and emotionally supportive figure even if some of these characteristics have a negative effect on patient compliance. These statements are controversial and may in part be explained by psychophysiological factors involved in health and disease. Relieving patients of their anxieties and fear of their condition can affect psychophysiological mechanisms which may result in a reduction in the experience of pain and autonomic reactions, and patients subsequently report a decrease in their symptoms (Adams et al 1993, Wyke 1987).

MAINTENANCE OF PROFESSIONALISM

The practitioner uses communication not only to convey information about the patient's condition and treatment, but also to establish roles and relations with the patient. The therapist establishes the role of professional by providing information and reassurance, listening to the patient and showing empathy with the patient. The difference between a professional relationship which appears to incorporate the qualities of friendship but is not a true friendship lies in the fact that the interaction is purely patient-oriented and only the patient's welfare is considered. It appears that a truly equal partnership is incongruous with professionalism and may cross social boundaries, which may not be advantageous to either patient or practitioner.

Davis (1968, 1971) found compliance with instructions to improve when both patient and doctor acted according to their roles and the socio-emotional factors were addressed satisfactorily. Therefore it appears that a paternal-type authority may be advantageous in the medical encounter and may in part explain the credence that patients attach to their male consultants in terms of establishing a mutual understanding about their medical condition.

It appears that when an encounter requires one party to undress, becoming physically and emotionally vulnerable, and be handled by the other party, the integrity of professionalism is maintained by adhering to strict social boundaries and acting largely to traditional roles of active practitioner participation with the patient as a passive recipient of care (Willson & McNamara 1982). These roles appear to be effective, providing adequate information is given to patients and they are involved in the management of their condition and understand the medical reasons for complying with instructions.

FACTORS AFFECTING HEALTH OUTCOMES

There are profound psychological factors affecting any therapeutic relationship. These factors are conveyed in the process of communication in the therapeutic encounter and affect health outcomes. Physiologically, the mechanisms involved in reducing cortical activity by relieving anxiety, fear and uncertainty by providing adequate reassurance and explanation are effected via the corticospinal and reticulospinal tracts synapsing in the spinal cord (Jayson 1987, Adams et al 1993). These may close the hypo-thetical 'gate' in the spinal cord to painful impulses (Melzack & Wall 1989) and thus the experience of pain is reduced.

Therefore these psychological factors in patient–practitioner interactions which are affected by the process of communication, may also influence physical outcomes of treatment.

It is argued that providing adequate information and reassurance and touching the patient are the most important components of communi-cation in the therapeutic encounter. It appears that the more information that is provided by the practitioner, the more likelihood there is of patient compliance.

By being included in the consultation and involved in the decision making, the patient should experience an increase in feelings of control of the situation which may relieve feelings of hopelessness and helpless-ness which, according to Seligman (1975), may contribute to feelings of depression and despair. If patients are not able to express their worries and fears, they are more likely, according to Havelock (1991), to consult again.

PSYCHOLOGICAL PREPARATION FOR TREATMENT

It is important to prepare patients psychologically for their treatment programmes as this will reduce their overall pain experience by giving them a feeling of control over their pain. This may be achieved by providing patients with information about what will happen during treatment, how this will feel and the consequences of the treatment. If the treatment is likely to be painful, this will provide patients with an understanding of why it is painful and how this will ultimately provide pain relief, e.g. a chronic back pain patient who has weakening and fibrosis due to misuse and underuse of the paraspinal soft tissues and has lost all range of movement in extension. When this person first performs extension procedures, this will be painful. However, if the person is prepared for this pain and understands that it will only occur until range of movement has been achieved, then he will not be afraid of damaging his back and will continue with his rehabilitation. The therapist must therefore explain this to the patient.

A number of experimental studies have demonstrated that the stress of electric shock and noxious stimuli is reduced if subjects are made aware in advance of the timing and intensity of shocks and if subjects are aware that there is no risk of injury. Turk et al (1983) developed a procedure for enhancing subjects' ability to control their response to painful stimuli and thus increase their pain tolerance. The subjects were instructed about the nature of the pain and asked to imagine the experience. Recommendations of how to cope with the pain were also provided. They were instructed to relax and trained to redirect and reinterpret the painful experience. During the experiment the subjects were told to hold a hand in ice-cold water for a maximum length of time. The experimental group managed to extend this length of time by 75% and also showed a significant decrease in pain ratings. Practitioners can use these techniques when instructing a patient during a painful procedure.

This evidence suggests that the distress associated with an unpleasant procedure can be reduced by making the patient aware of the procedure and its implications. It is necessary to provide reassurance to the patient that the procedure is beneficial and not harmful. It is also helpful to allow the patient to control the rate of progression, e.g. if a procedure becomes too painful, the patient raises a hand and the therapist will stop until the patient feels able to continue.

IMPLICATIONS FOR PRACTITIONERS

All practitioners, irrespective of their particular disciplines, in their inter-action with patients, are addressing psychological aspects of their patients' condition. It has been described how the signs and symptoms of depression include a feeling of loss of control and feelings of hopelessness and helplessness. These feelings are also experienced by chronic low back pain patients whose daily lives are affected by the incapacitating effects of their pain. Several studies discussed in previous chapters have suggested that any treatment programme for chronic low back pain should place emphasis on control by the patient in order that a pattern of hopelessness and helplessness does not emerge. Active patient participation may partially explain the success of these treatment programmes where patients assume responsibility for management of their own condition and control their own rate of progression.

The ideal treatment for chronic low back pain appears to be a combi-nation of physical and psychological intervention. Physiotherapists not only provide a physical treatment in correcting the biomechanical dys-function but also the interaction between patient and therapist may fulfil a psychological need in these patients. Various studies have suggested the need for chronic pain patients to be 'parented' into coping and managing their pain. Reassurance by practitioners that there is no serious underlying pathology, and clear explanation as to the possible reasons for pain, increases patients' understanding of their own condition and reduces anxiety, fear and uncertainty—which consequently reduces the experience of pain.

As discussed in previous chapters, reinforcement for positive behaviours and attitudes should be provided by therapists before patients assume a career in pain (Carron & McLaughlin 1982). A successful behaviour-modification programme has been established by Williams (1989) based on the principles of reinforcing well behaviours in chronic pain patients. Patients were encouraged to take responsibility for their own condition using the medium of physical activity. This returns the feeling of control of the situation to patients. This approach is also psychologically beneficial in addition to the obvious biomechanical effects of treatment and advice. It appears that these patients, who often have a history of caring for others, require a period of care for themselves in terms of both physical treatment and emotional support. It is a delicate balance between providing an adequate level of support for patients while encouraging responsibility and self-management to prevent patterns of illness behaviour and dependency emerging. As clinical consultations require patients to undress and be physically handled by practitioners, patients are frequently more likely to disclose personal information. If practitioners discover any histories of abuse, it is recommended that the patients also receive professional counselling.

Summary

There are a number of psychological factors in patient–practitioner interactions which may influence the process and outcomes of treatment. Communication is an integral part of the patient–practitioner relationship and is the most significant factor in influencing patient satisfaction or dissatisfaction with treatment.

Communication involves both verbal and nonverbal behaviours, such as provision of information, listening, empathy and use of touch. In addition to their treatment, it is important that patients feel that they have been listened to and experience a feeling of caring. Provision of information is important to ensure patient compliance and prepare patients for treatment; adequate preparation and explanation will reduce anxiety which can limit recovery.

It is argued that communication is as important as the treatment itself, and the practitioner in this way is a powerful mediator for improvement.

SUMMARY OF MAIN POINTS

1. The patient–practitioner interaction exerts a powerful effect on treatment outcomes. Appropriate interpersonal skills are therefore imperative for health professionals.

2. The qualities rated most highly in health professionals are listening, explaining adequately, spending time in the consultation and being caring.

3. Two types of behaviour are important in the medical consultation. These are:

   a. instrumental (task-oriented) behaviours such as providing information, questioning and directing the patient through the consultation

   b. affective behaviours, which refer to behaviours with an emotional content; these include showing concern and empathy.

4. Patients' needs for information include information about the nature and course of their illness, treatment plans, process and after effects of diagnostic and therapeutic procedures. Compliance is related to the level of appropriate information provided.

5. Empathy is usually communicated through nonverbal behaviours such as eye contact, body positioning, touch and voice tone.

6. Touch in therapeutic encounters may be used to examine and treat the patient's physical condition. However, it may also be used to convey reassurance and empathy.

7. The ideal treatment for CLBP appears to be a combination of physical and psychological intervention. The interaction between patient and practitioner may fulfil a psychological need in these patients and adequate preparation for treatment including explanation and reassurance will reduce anxiety and pain. Thus it is argued that communication is an important component of treatment and the patient-practitioner interaction is a powerful mediator for improvement.

10

Conclusions

Nicola Adams

Pain is a complex subjective experience that is mediated through multiple components of the peripheral and central nervous systems. It is made up of psychological, physiological and biochemical components which interact to produce the experience of pain. Pain may be modulated at various levels of the neuraxis and is influenced not only by nociceptive impulses from areas of tissue damage, but also by psychological factors such as anxiety, past experience of pain, and socially and culturally learned interpretations and responses to pain. In chronic pain conditions, there may also be involvement of neurochemical factors which may not only contribute to the experience of pain but also to associated autonomic and psychological responses. The majority of chronic low back pain patients demonstrate physiological dysfunction with contributory psychological and behavioural dysfunction, and thus the potential for these patients to respond to a wide variety of interventions is great.

IMPLICATIONS FOR PRACTITIONERS

Psychological factors ultimately determine the patient's perception and response to pain. It is important for any practitioner to address psychological factors in the pain experience, as addressing these will have a profound effect on the outcome of treatment. Psychological factors that are important in low back pain include personality factors, cognitive factors such as ability to cope, and behavioural factors such as illness behaviour. The social and cultural background, beliefs and expectations of the patient should be taken into consideration, as these will affect the approach selected by the practitioner.

Directions in practice

Patients are encouraged to take greater responsibility for their health and well-being and thus the management of their own condition. Treatment for low back pain has thus progressed from symptomatic treatment provided by the practitioner to education and self-management in which patients are viewed as active participants in the process of treatment. An increasing number of back management programmes based on psychological principles have emerged, though their efficacy has yet to be scientifically evaluated.

Use of psychological approaches

Psychological techniques can be used by psychologists in the treatment of low back pain. However, any practitioners may incorporate psychological approaches in their treatment, even if their discipline is not psychology. Psychological approaches are often based on a cognitive–behavioural model, where the patients' illness behaviours are not reinforced whereas well behaviours are positively reinforced. Goal-setting and education may increase patients' feelings of control over their condition, and reassurance given by the practitioner may reduce anxiety and thus pain. The psychological approach used may also influence outcomes of treatment and augment physical treatment.

The patient–practitioner interaction

Despite an emphasis on control and self-management, there is an interesting paradox in the power of the practitioner in the interaction with patients. In the treatment process, this power of the patient–practitioner relationship should not be underestimated, as it has considerable power to define outcomes of treatment. This may be attributed to a placebo effect, suggestion, patient expectations or a feeling of control in having professional attention. Recent research has suggested that a transfer of energy between two persons may occur, particularly where therapeutic touch is involved. According to this theory, which is based on Eastern medicine, the practitioner transfers some of his or her own energy to the patient whose energy levels have been blocked or depleted. There are many avenues for exploration in this area.

Use of touch

Touch is one of the most influential components of the therapeutic encounter as it carries profound and varied meanings and interpretations. There are two main purposes of touch in the therapeutic encounter; the first is to examine or perform a treatment procedure and the second, equally important, function is to reassure and convey empathy. Patients are more likely to confide in the practitioner whose treatment involves touch. Many chronic pain patients have a subconscious need for reassuring (non-sexual) touch and the practitioner may in some way fulfil this need without the emotional connotations ordinarily associated with this action.

RECOMMENDATIONS

A number of recommendations can be made on the basis of the research reviewed in this text.

Detection of patients at risk

The use of short psychological tests may indicate which patients may be at risk for developing chronic pain. The practitioner may thus be able to incorporate an appropriate approach to treatment in the early stages. This may also assist with the problem of referral in providing some guidelines to medical practitioners as to which patient may benefit from physiotherapy and which patient would be better treated by a psychologist, social worker or orthopaedic surgeon.

Diagnostic criteria

The use of the standardized examination procedures may assist in diagnosis in order that appropriate treatment may be implemented. Differential diagnosis should lead to differential treatment. Electromyography may have uses in providing objective measures to confirm clinical diagnosis and this may be useful in litigation cases.

A future direction in research is the use of neuropeptides as a diagnostic aid in chronic pain; however, research in this area is yet in its infancy.

Quantification of outcome measures

Electromyography is often used as a diagnostic tool and it is also used in biofeedback treatment. However, another important use of EMG is to quantify outcome measures. EMG analysis can provide an objective assessment of the biomechanical response to treatment, and the patient is unable to falsify this information. Thus EMG may be useful as an objective measure in the evaluation of practice.

There is a growing awareness of psychological factors in low back pain, and indeed in many illnesses. There are significant psychological factors in low back pain; however, there are also significant physiological and biochemical factors. Which factors are causes of low back pain and which its result is largely unknown. It is hoped that this book, rather than providing answers, has stimulated ideas for both practice and research into this difficult but prevalent condition.

References

Adams N B K 1986 Psychological aspects of chronic low back pain. Unpublished undergraduate research. University of Ulster, Coleraine.

Adams N B K 1992 Psychophysiological and neurochemical substrates of chronic low back pain and modulation by treatment. Doctoral dissertation, University of Ulster, Coleraine

Adams N, Ravey J, Bell A J 1993 An investigation of electromyographic assessment of treatment outcomes following a standardised treatment programme for chronic low back pain patients. Proceedings of the 24th Annual Meeting of the Association for Applied Psychophysiology and Biofeedback, Los Angeles, California

Adams N, Ravey J, Bell J 1994 A review of personality characteristics in chronic low back pain. Physiotherapy 80: 511–513

Adams N, Whittington D, Saunders C, Bell J 1994 Communication skills in physiotherapist–patient interactions. University of Ulster, Coleraine

Ahern D, Follick M 1985 Distress in spouses of chronic pain patients. International Journal of Family Therapy 7: 247

Ahern D K, Follick M J 1988 Comparison of lumbar paravertebral EMG patterns in chronic low back pain patients and non-patient controls. Pain 34: 153–160

Ahles T A, Yunus M B, Masi A T 1987 Is chronic pain a variant of depressive disease? The case of primary fibromyalgia syndrome. Pain 29: 105–111

Ahrens S, Deffner G 1986 Empirical study of alexithymia: methodology and results. American Journal of Psychotherapy 40: 430–447

Alexander A 1975 An experimental test of assumptions relating to the use of EMG biofeedback as a general relaxation training technique. Psychophysiology 12: 656–662

Almay B G L, Johansson F, von Knorring L, Le Greves P, Terenius L 1988 Substance P in CSF of patients with chronic pain syndromes. Pain 33: 3–9

American Psychiatric Association 1987 American Diagnostic and Statistical Manual of Mental Disorders (DSM-IV). American Psychiatric Association, Washington DC

Andersson G B J 1981 Epidemiological aspects of low back pain in industry. Spine 6: 53–60

Andrasik F, Holroyd K A 1980 A test of specific and non specific effects in the biofeedback treatment of tension headache. Journal of Consulting and Clinical Psychology 48: 575–586

Appley M H, Trumbull R 1986 The dynamics of stress: physiological, psychological and social perspectives. Plenum Press, New York

Arena J G, Sherman R A, Bruno G M, Young T R 1991 Electromyographic recordings of low back pain subjects and non pain controls in six different positions. Pain 45: 23–28

Arnetz B B, Fjellner B 1986 Psychological predictors of neuroendocrine responses to mental stress. Journal of Psychosomatic Research 30: 297–305

Aronin N, Difiglia M, Leeman S E 1983 Substance P. In: Krieger D T, Brownstein M J, Martin J B (eds) Brain peptides. John Wiley, New York

Asfour S S, Ayoub M M 1984 Effects of an endurance strength training programme on lifting capabilities of males. Ergonomics 27: 435–442

Ashton I K, Ashton B A, Gibson S J, Polak J M, Jaffrey D C 1992 Morphological basis for back pain: the demonstration of nerve fibres and neuropeptides in the lumbar facet joint capsule but not in ligamentum flavum. Journal of Orthopaedic Research 10: 72–78

Atweh S F, Kuhar M J 1977 Audiographic localisation of opiate receptors in the rat brain: 1. Spinal cord and lower medulla. Brain Research 124: 5

Averill J R, Opton E M Jr, Lazarus R S 1969 Cross-cultural studies of psychophysiological responses during stress and emotion. International Journal of Psychology 4: 83–102

Bain D 1976 Doctor–patient communication in general practice consultations. Medical Education 10: 125–131

Baker G H B 1987 Invited review. Psychological factors and immunity. Journal of Psychosomatic Research 31: 1–10

Baldessarini R J 1975 Drugs and the treatment of psychiatric disorders. In: Gilman A G, Goodman L S, Rall T W, Murad F (eds) The pharmacological basis of therapeutics, 7th edn. Macmillan Press, New York

Balint M 1964 The doctor, his patient and the illness. Pitman, London

Bandura A 1977 Self efficacy: towards a unifying theory of behavioural change. Psychological Review 84: 191–215

Basbaum A I 1985 Functional analysis of the cytochemistry of the spinal dorsal horn. In: Fields H L, Dubner R, Gervero F (eds) Advances in pain research and therapy. Raven Press, New York, vol IX

Basbaum A I, Fields H L 1984 Endogenous pain control systems: brainstem spinal pathways and endorphin circuitry. Annual Reviews in Neuroscience 7: 309–338

Basbaum A I, Fields H L 1978 Endogenous pain control mechanisms. Review and hypothesis. Annals of Neurology 4: 451

Basmajian J V 1983 Biofeedback principles and practice for clinicians, 2nd edn. Williams & Wilkins, Baltimore

Bates J A V, Nathan P W 1980 Transcutaneous electrical nerve stimulation for chronic pain. Anaesthesia 35: 817–822

Beck A 1984 Cognitive approaches to stress. In: Woolfolk R L, Lehrer P M (eds) Principles and practice of stress management. Guilford Press, New York, pp 255–305

Beecher H K 1959 Measurement of subjective pain responses. Oxford University Press, Oxford

Bellack A S, Hersen M, Kazdin A E 1982 International handbook of behaviour modification and therapy. Plenum Press, New York

Bellissimo A, Turks E 1984 Chronic pain: the psychotherapeutic spectrum. Praeger, New York

Bengston R 1983 Physical measures useful in pain management. International Anaesthesiology. Clinics in Pain Management 21: 165–176

Bennett T L 1977 Brain and behaviour. Brook Cole, California

Bensing J M, Dronkers J 1992 Instrumental and affective aspects of physician behaviour. Medical Care 30: 283–298

Benson H 1975 The relaxation response. Morrow, New York

Benson H 1977 Systemic hypertension and the relaxation response. New England Journal of Medicine 296: 1152–1156

Benson H, McCallie D P 1979 Angina pectoris and the placebo effect. New England Journal of Medicine 300: 1424–1429

Benson H, Rosner B A, Marzetta B, Klemchuk H 1974 Decreased blood pressure in pharmacologically treated hypertensive patients who regularly elicited the relaxation response. Lancet i: 289–292

Bernstein D A, Borkovek T D 1973 Progressive relaxation training. Research Press Champaign, Ill

Bernstein D A, Given B A 1984 Progressive relaxation: abbreviated methods. In: Woolfolk R L, Lehrer P M (eds) Principles and practice of stress management. Guilford Press, New York, pp 43–69

Bessou P, Perl E R 1969 Response of cutaneous sensory units with unmyelinated fibres to noxious stimuli. Journal of Neurophysiology 39: 1160

Bigos S J, Spengler D M, Martin N A, Zeh J, Fisher L, Nachemson A 1986 Back injuries in industry: a retrospective study. III. Employee related factors. Spine 11: 252–256

Bishop B 1980 Pain: physiology and rationale for management. Physical Therapy 60: 13–27

Black R G 1975 The chronic pain syndrome. Surgical Clinics of North America 55: 999

Bloch R 1987 Methodology in clinical back pain trials. Spine 12: 430–432

Block A R 1981 An investigation of the response of the spouse to chronic pain behaviour. Psychosomatic Medicine 4: 425–432

Blumer D, Heilbronn M 1982 Chronic pain as a variant of depressive disease. Journal of Nervous and Mental Diseases 170: 381–395

Blumer D, Heilbronn M, Rosenbaum A H 1982 Antidepressant treatment of the pain prone disorder. Psychopharmacological Bulletin 20: 531–535

Bombardier C, Kerr M S, Shannon H S, Frank J W 1994 A guide to interpreting epidemiologic studies on the etiology of back pain. Spine 19: 2047S–2056S

Bond M 1984 Pain: its nature, analysis and treatment. Churchill Livingstone, Edinburgh

Bonica J J 1990 Management of pain. Lea & Febiger, Philadelphia, vols I, II

Boreham P, Gibson D 1978 The informative process in private medical consultations: a preliminary investigation. Social Science and Medicine 12: 409–415

Borenstein D G, Weisel S W, Boden S D 1995 Low back pain: medical diagnosis and comprehensive management. W B Saunders, Philadelphia

Borkovek T D, Grayson, J B, Cooper K M 1978 Treatment of general tension: subjective and physiological effects of progressive relaxation. Journal of Consulting and Clinical Psychology 46: 518–528

Bowsher D 1988 Introduction to anatomy and physiology of the nervous system. Blackwell Scientific Publications, Oxford

Boyle C M 1970 Differences between patients and doctors interpretations of some common medical terms. British Medical Journal 2: 286–289

Bradish C F, Lloyd G J, Adam C H, Albert J, Dyson P, Doxey N C S, Mitson G L 1988 Do nonorganic signs help to predict the return to activity of patients with low back pain? Spine 13: 557–560

Bradley L A, McCreary C, Williams D A 1993 MMPI and personality assessment instruments: useful in evaluating chronic pain patients. Abstracts of the 7th World Congress on Pain. IASP Press, Seattle, p 356

Brady J V 1970 Endocrine and autonomic correlates of emotional behaviour. In: Black P (ed) Physiological correlates of emotion. Academic Press, New York

Brimijohn S 1980 Axonal transport of substance P in the vagus and sciatic nerves of the guinea pig. Brain Research 191: 443

Brody D S 1980 An analysis of patient recall of their therapeutic regimes. Journal of Chronic Diseases 33: 57–62

Brown B 1977 Stress and the art of biofeedback. Harper & Row, New York

Buchanan J 1991 Doctor–patient communication. New Zealand Medical Journal 104: 62–64

Budzynski T H, Stoyva J M 1984 Biofeedback methods in the treatment of anxiety and stress. In: Woolfolk R L, Lehrer P M (eds) Principles and practice of stress management. Guilford Press, New York, pp 188–219

Burgess P R, Perl E R 1973 Cutaneous mechanoreceptors and nociceptors. In: Iggo A (ed) Handbook of sensory physiology Vol 2. Somatosensory system. Springer-Verlag, Berlin, p 9

Burish T G, Carey M P, Wallston K A, Stein M J, Jamison R N, Lyles J N 1984 Health locus of control and chronic disease: an external orientation may be advantageous. Journal of Social and Clinical Psychology 2: 326–332

Bush C, Ditto B 1985 A controlled evaluation of paraspinal EMG biofeedback in the treatment of chronic low back pain. Health Psychology 4: 307–321

Caldwell A, Chase C 1977 Diagnosis and treatment of personality factors in chronic low back pain. Clinical Orthopaedics and Related Research 129: 141–149

Cannon W B 1953 Bodily changes in pain, hunger, fear and rage. Charles T Branford, Boston

Capper S J 1986 Peptides in body fluids in pain. Progress in Brain Research 66: 317–30

Capra P, Mayer T G, Gatchel R 1985 Adding psychological scales to your back pain assessment. Journal of Musculoskeletal Medicine 2: 41–52

Carey M P, Burish T G 1985 Anxiety as a predictor of behavioral therapy outcome for cancer chemotherapy patients. Journal of Consulting and Clinical Psychology 53: 860–865

Carey M P, Burish T G 1987 Providing relaxation training to cancer chemotherapy patients: a comparison of three methods. Journal of Consulting and Clinical Psychology 55: 732–737

Carey M P, Burish T G 1988 Etiology and treatment of the psychological side effects associated with cancer chemotherapy: a critical review and discussion. Psychological Bulletin 104: 307–325

Carpenter M B, Stein B M, Shriver J E 1968 Central projections of spinal and dorsal roots in the monkey. II. Lower thoracic, lumbosacral and coccygeal dorsal roots. American Journal of Anatomy 123: 75

Carrington P 1984 Modern forms of meditation. In: Woolfolk R L, Lehrer P M (eds) Principles and practice of stress management. Guilford Press, New York, pp 108–141

Carrington P, Collings G H, Benson H, Robinson H, Wood L W, Lehrer P M, Woolfolk R L, Cole J W 1980 The use of meditation–relaxation techniques for the management of stress in a working population. Journal of Occupational Medicine 22: 221–231

Carron H, McLaughlin R E 1982 Management of low back pain. John Wright, Bristol

Cartwright A 1964 Human relations and hospital care. Routledge, London

Cassileth B R 1980 Information and participation preferences among cancer patients. Annals of Internal Medicine 92: 832–836

Cattell R B 1973 Personality and mood by questionnaire. Jossey-Bass, San Francisco

Cesselin F, Laporte A M, Miquel M C, Bourgoin S, Hamson M 1993 Serotonergic mechanisms of pain control. In: Gebhart G F, Hammond D L, Jensen T S (eds) Proceedings of the 7th World Congress on Pain. Progress in pain research and management, Vol 2. IASP Press, Seattle

Chan A C N, Chapman C R 1980 Aspirin analgesia evaluated by event related potentials in man: possible central actions in the brain. Experimental Brain Research 39: 359–364

Chang M M, Leeman S E, Niall H D 1971 Amino acid sequence of substance P. Nature New Biology 232: 86–87

Charman R 1989 Pain theory and physiotherapy. Physiotherapy 75: 247–254

China Sports 1984 How the 'wild goose' breathing exercise cures. China Sports 10: 43–48; 11: 55–59; 12: 58–60; appendix

Christie M J, Mellett P G 1981 Foundations of psychosomatics. John Wiley, Chichester

Christie M J, Mellett P G 1986 The psychosomatic approach. Contemporary practice of whole person care. John Wiley, Chichester

Chudler E H, Dong W K 1995 The role of the basal ganglia in nociception and pain. Pain 60: 3–37

Ciccone D S, Grzesiak R C 1984 Cognitive dimensions of chronic pain. Social Science and Medicine 19: 1339–1345

Cicourel A 1981 Language and medicine. In: Ferguson C A, Health S B (eds) Language in the USA. Cambridge University Press, New York, p 407–429

Clinical Standards Advisory Group (CSAG) 1994 Report of the CSAG Committee on back pain HMSO

Coggeshall R E 1979 Afferent fibres in the ventral root. Neurosurgery 4: 443

Collet L, Cottraux J, Juenet C 1986 Tension headaches: relationship between MMPI paranoia score and MMPI hypochondriasis score and frontalis EMG. Headache 26: 365–368

Collins G A, Cohen M J 1982 A comparative analysis of paraspinal and frontalis EMG, heart rate and conductance in chronic low back pain patients and normals to various postures and stresses. Scandinavian Journal of Rehabilitation Medicine 14: 39–46

Copeman W 1969 Textbook of rheumatic diseases. Churchill Livingstone, Edinburgh

Cott A, Anchel H, Goldberg W M, Fabich M, Parkinson W 1990 Non-institutional treatment of chronic pain by field management: an outcome study with comparison group. Pain 40: 183–194

Cox T 1981 Stress. Macmillan Press, London

Cox T, Mackay C 1982 Psychosocial factors and psychophysiological mechanisms in the aetiology and development of cancers. Social Science and Medicine 16: 381–396

Craig K D 1978 Social modeling influences on pain. In: Sternbach R A (ed) The psychology of pain. Raven Press, New York, pp 73–79

Cram J R 1990 Clinical EMG for surface recordings. Clinical Resources, Nevada City, vol II

Cram J R, Steger J C 1983 EMG scanning in the diagnosis of chronic pain. Biofeedback and Self Regulation 8: 229–241

Croft J J 1980 Interviewing in physical therapy. Physical Therapy 60: 1033–1036

Cromin R E, Erikson A M, deTorrente A 1978 Norepinephrine induced acute renal failure. Kidney International 14: 187–190

Crown S 1978 Psychological aspects of low back pain. Rheumatology and Rehabilitation 17: 114

Cuello A C, Matthews M R 1989 Peptides in peripheral sensory nerve fibres. In: Wall P D, Melzack R (eds) Textbook of pain. Churchill Livingstone, Edinburgh, pp 65–79

Culberson J L, Haines D E, Kimmel D L, Brown P B 1979 Contralateral projection of primary afferent fibres to mammalian spinal cord. Experimental Neurology 64: 83

Cyriax J. 1984 Textbook of orthopaedic medicine, Vol 2. Balliere Tindall, London

Daly E J, Donn P A, Galliher M J, Zimmerman J S 1983 Biofeedback applications to migraine and tension headaches: A double-blinded outcome study. Biofeedback and Self-Regulation 8: 135–152

Damkot D K, Pope M H, Lord J, Frymoyer J W 1984 The relationship between work history, work environment and low back pain in men. Spine 9: 395–399

Dansak D 1973 On the tertiary gain of illness. Comprehensive Psychiatry 14: 523

Danton W G, May J R, Lynn E J 1984 Psychological and physiological effects of relaxation and nitrous oxide training. Psychological Reports 55: 311–322

Davidson D M, Winchester M A, Taylor C B, Alderman E A, Ingels N B 1979 Effects of relaxation therapy on cardiac performance and sympathetic activity in patients with organic heart disease. Psychosomatic Medicine 41: 303–309

Davis M S 1966 Variations in patients compliance with doctors orders: analysis of the congruence between survey responses and results of empirical investigations. Journal of Medical Education 41: 1037

Davis M S 1968 Variations in patient compliance with doctors advice: an empirical analysis of patterns. American Journal of Public Health 58: 274

Davis M S 1971 Variation in patients compliance with doctors orders: medical practice and doctor–patient interaction. Psychiatric Medicine 2: 31

De Domenico G 1982 Pain relief with interferential therapy. Australian Journal of Physiotherapy 28: 14–18

Devlin T M 1986 Textbook of biochemistry with clinical correlations, 2nd edn. John Wiley, New York

Deyo R A 1983 Conservative therapy for low back pain. Journal of the American Medical Association 250: 1057–1062

Dickson D A, Hargie O D W, Morrow N C 1989, Communication skills training for health professionals: an instructors handbook. Chapman and Hall, London

Dickson D A, Maxwell M 1987 A comparative study of physiotherapy students attitudes to social skills training before and after clinical placement. Physiotherapy 73: 60–64

Dillard J, Trafimow J, Anderson B J, Cronin K 1991 Motion of the lumbar spine. Reliability of two measurement techniques. Spine 16: 321–324

Dimaggio A, Mooney V 1987 The McKenzie program: exercise effective against back pain. Journal of Musculoskeletal Medicine (Dec): 63–72

DiMatteo M R 1979 A social-psychological analysis of physician patient rapport: toward a science of the art of medicine. Journal of Social Science 35: 12

Dixon A St J 1973 Progress and problems in back pain research. Rheumatology and Rehabilitation 12: 165–174

Doan B D, Wadden P 1989 Relationships between depressive symptoms and descriptions of chronic pain. Pain 36: 75–84

Donaldson S, Donaldson M 1990 Multichannel EMG assessment and treatment techniques. In: Cram J R (ed) Clinical EMG for surface recordings. Clinical Resources, Nevada City, vol II

Dorian B, Garfinkel P, Brown G, Shore A, Gladman D, Keystone E 1982 Aberrations in lymphocyte subpopulations and function during psychological stress. Clinical and Experimental Immunology 50: 132–138

Dubner R, Bennett C J 1983 Spinal and trigeminal mechanisms of nociception. Annual Review of Neuroscience 6: 381

Dubner R, Sumino R, Wood W I 1975 A peripheral 'cold' fibre population responsive to innocuous and noxious thermal stimuli applied to the monkeys face. Journal of Neurophysiology 38: 1373

Dworkin R H, Richlin D M, Handlin D S, Brand L 1986 Predicting treatment response in depressed and non-depressed chronic pain patients. Pain 24: 343–353

Echternach J 1987 Pain. Clinics in physical therapy Vol 12. Churchill Livingstone, New York

Eisenberg D 1985 Encounters with Qi: understanding Chinese medicine. Norton, New York

Elton D, Stanley G, Burrows C 1983 Psychological control of pain. Grune & Stratton, Australia

Engel G 1959 Psychogenic pain and the pain prone patient. American Journal of Medicine 26: 899–918

Engel G L 1988 How much longer must medicines science be bound by a seventeenth century world view? In: White K (ed) The task of medicine. The Henry J Kaiser Family Foundation, Menlo Park, CA

Erpsamer V 1981 The tachykinin peptide family. Trends in Neuroscience 4: 267–269

Erpsamer V, Melchiorri P 1980 Active polypeptides from amphibian skin to gastrointestinal tracts and brains of mammals. Trends in Pharmacological Science 1: 391–393

Evarts E V 1975 Activity of motor cortex neurons in association with learned movement. International Journal of Neuroscience 3: 113–124

Eysenck H J, Eysenck S B G 1975 Manual of the Eysenck Personality Questionnaire. Hodder & Stoughton, Kent

Fairbank J C T, Couper J, Davies J B, O'Brien J P 1980 The Oswestry Low Back Pain Disability Questionnaire. Physiotherapy 66: 271–273

Ferreira S H, Vane J R 1974 New aspects of the mode of action of non-steroid anti-inflammatory drugs: Annual Review of Pharmacology 14: 57

Fields H L 1985 Neural mechanisms of opiate analgesia. In: Fields H L, Dubner R, Cervero F (eds) Advances in pain research and therapy. Raven Press, New York, vol IX

Finneson B E 1980 Low back pain. Lippincott, Philadelphia Flint C 1988 Know your midwife. Nursing Times 84: 28–32

Flor H, Haag, Turk D C 1980 Efficacy of EMG biofeedback, pseudotherapy and conventional medical treatment for chronic rheumatic back pain. Pain 17: 21–31

Flor H, Birbaumer N, Schulte W, Roos R 1991 Stress related electromyographic responses in patients with chronic temperomandibular pain. Journal of Chronic Diseases 21: 21, 179–190

Flor H, Turk D, Rudy T 1987 Pain and families II. Assessment and treatment. Pain 30: 29

Floyd W F, Silver P 1955 The functions of the erector spinae muscles in certain movements and postures in man. Journal of Physiology 129: 184–203

Folkow B, Gothberg G, Lundin S 1977 Structural resetting of the renal vascular bed in spontaneously hypertensive rats. Acta Physiologica Scandinavica 100: 270–272

Follick M J, Smith T W, Ahern D K 1985 The sickness impact profile: a global measure of disability in chronic low back pain. Pain 21: 61–76

Fordyce W E 1976 Behavioural methods for chronic pain and illness. C V Mosby, St Louis

Fordyce W E 1979 Environmental factors in the genesis of low back pain. In: Bonica J J, Liebeskind J E, Albe Fessard D G (eds) Proceedings of the 2nd World Congress on Pain. Advances in Pain Research and Therapy. Raven Press, New York, vol 3

Fordyce W E 1986 Learning processes in pain. In: Sternbach R A (ed) The psychology of pain. Raven Press, New York

Fordyce W E, Fowler R S, Lehman J F, De Lateur B J 1968 Some implications of learning in problems of chronic pain. Journal of Chronic Diseases 21: 179–190

Fordyce W E, Fowler R S, Lehman J F, DeLateur B J, Sand P L, Treischmann R 1973 Operant conditioning in the treatment of chronic pain: Archives of Physical Medicine and Rehabilitation 54: 399–408

Foreman R D, Schmidt R F, Willis W D 1979 Effects of mechanical and chemical stimulation of fine muscle afferents upon primate spinothalamic tract cells. Journal of Physiology 286: 215

Forrest A J, Wolkind S N 1974 Masked depression in men with low back pain. Rheumatology and Rehabilitation 13: 148–153

France R D, Krishnan K R, Trainor M 1986 Chronic pain and depression. III. Family history of depression and alcoholism in CLBP patients. Pain 24: 185–190

Francis V, Korsch B M, Morris M J 1969 Gaps in doctor patient communication. Patients' response to medical advice. New England Journal of Medicine 280: 535–540

Freeman C, Calsyn C 1980 Biofeedback with low back pain patients. American Journal of Clinical Biofeedback 3: 118–122

Freeman C, Calsyn D, Louks J 1976 The use of the MMPI with low back pain patients. Journal of Clinical Psychology 32: 294–298

French S 1989 Pain: some psychological and sociological aspects. Physiotherapy 75: 255–260

French S 1992 Physiotherapy. A psychosocial approach. Butterworth Heinemann, Oxford

Friedman M, Rosenman R 1974 Type A behaviour and your heart. Wildwood House, London

Friedson E 1970 Professional dominance. Aldine, Chicago

Frymoyer J W, Pope M H, Clements J H, Wilder D G, MacPherson B, Ashikaga T 1983 Risk factors in low back pain: an epidemiological survey. Journal of Bone and Joint Surgery 65A: 213–218

Gamble R P, Stevens A B, McBrien H, Black A, Boreham C A G 1991 Physical fitness and occupational demands of the Belfast ambulance service. British Journal of Industrial Medicine 48: 592–596

Gamsa A 1994 The role of psychological factors in chronic pain. A half century of study. Pain 57: 5–15

Ganong W F 1995 Review of medical physiology. Prentice Hall, London

Gebhart G F, Sandkuhler J, Thalhammer J G, Zimmerman M 1983 Inhibition of spinal nociceptive information by stimulation in the midbrain of the cat is blocked by lidocaine microinjected in nucleus raphe magnus and medullary reticular formation. Journal of Neurophysiology 50: 1446–1448

Gil K M, Ross S L, Keefe F J 1988 Behavioral treatment of chronic pain. Four management protocols. In: France R D, Krishnan K D D (eds) Chronic pain. American Psychiatric Press, Washington, pp 376–413

Gill K, Krag H, Johnson G B, Hough L D, Pope M H 1988 Repeatability of four clinical methods for assessment of lumbar spinal motion. Spine 13: 50–53

Gilman A G, Nall T W, Nies A S, Taylor P 1991 Pharmacological basis of therapeutics. McGraw Hill, New York

Goffman E 1961 Encounters: two studies in the sociology of interaction. Bobbs-Merrill, Indianapolis

Golden J S, Johnston G D 1970 Problems of distortion in doctor–patient communication. Psychiatric Medicine 1: 127

Goldstein D S, Dionne R, Sweet J, Gracely R, Brewer H B, Gregg R, Keiser H R 1982 Circulatory, plasma catecholamine, cortisol, lipid and psychological responses to a real-life stress (third molar extractions): effects of diazepam sedation and of inclusion of epinephrine with local anaesthetic. Psychosomatic Medicine 44: 259–272

Goldstein G, Hersen M 1984 Handbook of psychological assessment. Pergamon Press, New York

Grabel J A 1973 Electromyographic study of low back muscle tension in subjects with and without chronic low back pain. Dissertation Abstracts International 34: (6-B) 2929–2930

Grant D 1979 The physiotherapist as patient counsellor Physiotherapy 65: 218–220

Gray J A 1985 Issues in the neuropsychology of anxiety. In: Tuma A H, Maser J D (eds) Anxiety and anxiety disorders. Erlbaum, New Jersey

Grieve G P 1991 Mobilisation of the spine. Churchill Livingstone, Edinburgh

Grzesiak R C, Perrine K R 1987 Psychological aspects of chronic pain. In: Wu W H, Smith R G (eds) Pain management. Assessment of chronic and acute syndromes. Human Sciences Press, New York, pp 44–69

Gunn C 1989 Neuropathic pain. A new theory for chronic pain of intrinsic origin. Annals of the Royal College of Physicians and Surgeons Canada 22: 327–330

Guyton A C 1986 Textbook of medical physiology. W B Saunders, Philadelphia

Halliday A M, Logue V 1972 Painful sensations evoked by electrical stimulation in the thalamus. In: Somjen G G (ed) Neurophysiology studied in man. Excerpta Medica, Amsterdam, p 2210

Hamilton-Duckett P, Kidd L 1985 Counselling skills and the physiotherapist. Physiotherapy 71: 179–180

Hammond D L 1985 Pharmacology of central pain-modulating networks (biogenic amines and non-opioid analgesics). In: Fields H L, Dubner R, Cervero F (eds) Advances in pain research and therapy. Raven Press, New York, vol IX

Hammond D L 1986 Control systems for nociceptive afferent processing: the descending inhibitory pathways. In: Yaksh T L (ed) Spinal afferent processing. Plenum Press, New York

Hancock M B, Rigamonti D D, Bryan R N 1973 Convergence in the lumbar spinal cord of pathways activated by splanchnic nerve and hindlimb cutaneous nerve stimulation. Experimental Neurology 38: 377

Harding V, C de C Williams A 1995 Extending physiotherapy skills using a psychological approach. Cognitive behavioural management of chronic pain. Physiotherapy 81: 681–688

Harper R G, Steger J C 1978 Psychological correlates of frontalis EMG and pain in tension headaches. Headache 18: 215–218

Hathaway S H, McKinley J C 1969 The MMPI. University of Minnesota Press, Minneapolis

Havelock P 1991 Improving consultation skills. Practitioner 235–238

Haythornthwaite J A, Sieber W J, Kerns R D 1991 Depression and the chronic pain experience. Pain 46: 177–184

Headley B 1990 Comprehensive evaluation of postural dysfunction. Paper presented at 21st Annual Meeting of AAPB, Washington, DC

Hendler N, Derogatis L 1977 EMG biofeedback in patients with chronic pain. Diseases of the Nervous System 38: 505–509

Heszen-Klemens I, Lapinska E 1984 Doctor–patient interaction. Patients health behaviour and effects of treatment. Social Science and Medicine 19: 9–18

Hillenberg J B, Collins F L 1982 A procedural analysis and review of relaxation training research. Behavior Research and Therapy 20: 251–260

Hoffman J W, Benson H, Arns P A, Stainbrook G L, Landsberg L, Young J B, Gill A 1982 Reduced sympathetic nervous system responsivity associated with the relaxation response. Science 251: 190–192

Hokfelt T 1983 Neuropeptides and pain pathways. In: Bonica J J, Lindblom U, Iggo A (ed) Advances in pain research and therapy. Raven Press, New York, vol V

Holmes T H, Wolff H G 1952 Life situations, emotions and backache. Psychosomatic Medicine 14: 18–33

Holzman A D, Turk D C 1986. Pain management. A handbook of psychological treatment approaches. Pergamon Press, New York

Horal J 1969 The clinical appearance of low back disorders in the City of Gothenberg, Sweden. Acta Orthopaedica Scandinavica Supplementum 118: 1–109

Hoyt W H, Hunt H H 1981 EMG assessment of the chronic low back pain syndrome. Journal of the American Osteopathic Association 80: 57–59

Hughes J 1975 Identification of two related pentapeptides from the brain with potent opiate antagonist activity. Nature 258: 577

Hulka B S, Cassel J C, Kupper L L, Burdette J A 1976 Communication, compliance and concordance between physicians and patients with prescribed medications. American Journal of Public Health 66: 847

Huskisson E C 1974 Measurement of pain. Lancet 2: 1127–1131

Iggo A 1973 Handbook of sensory physiology. Vol 2: Somatosensory system. Springer-Verlag, Berlin

Iggo A 1960. Cutaneous mechanoreceptors with afferent C fibres. Journal of Physiology (London) 152: 337

Jacobsen E 1944 Progressive relaxation: a physiological and clinical investigation of muscular states and their significance in psychology and medical practice. University of Chicago Press, Chicago

Jacobson E 1938 Progressive relaxation. University of Chicago Press, Chicago

Jacobson E 1970 Modern treatment of tense patients. Charles C Thomas, Chicago

Jayson M I V 1987 The lumbar spine and back pain. Pitman Medical, Kent

Jayson M I V 1981 Back pain. The facts. Oxford Publications, Oxford

Johnson H E, Hockersmith V 1983 Therapeutic electromyography in chronic back pain. In: Basmajian J V (ed) Biofeedback principles and practice for clinicians Williams & Wilkins, Baltimore, pp 306–310

Karasu T B, Bellack L 1980 Specialised techniques in individual psychotherapy. Brunner/Mazel, New York

Keefe F J, Dunsmore J 1992a Pain behavior: concepts and controversies. American Pain Society Journal 1: 92–100

Keefe F J, Dunsmore J 1992b The multifaceted nature of pain behavior. American Pain Society Journal 1: 122–114

Keefe F J, Lefebvre J 1994 Pain behavior concepts: controversies, current status and future directions. Proceedings of 7th World Congress on Pain. In: Gebhart G F, Hammond D L, Jensen T S (eds) Progress in pain research and management. IASP Press, Seattle, vol 2

Keefe F J, Shapira B 1981 EMG assisted relaxation training in the management of chronic low back pain. American Journal of Clinical Biofeedback 4: 93–103

Keefe F J, Williams D A 1992 Assessment of pain behaviors. In: Turk D C, Melzack R (eds) Handbook of pain assessment. Guilford Press, New York, pp 275–294

Keefe F J, Block A R, Williams R B, Surwit R S 1981 Behavioral treatment of chronic low back pain: Clinical outcome and individual differences in pain relief. Pain 11: 221–231

Keefe F J, Wilkins R H, Cook W A 1984 Direct observation of pain behavior in low back pain patients during physical examination. Pain 20: 59–68

Keefe F J, Wilkins R H, Cook W A, Crisson J E, Mulbhaier L H 1986 Depression, pain and pain behaviour. Journal of Consulting Clinical Psychology 54: 665–669

Keele C A, Armstrong D 1964 Substances producing pain and itch. In: Barcroft H, Davson H, Paton W D M (eds) Monographs of the Physiological Society. Edward Arnold, London, vol XII, pp 1–374

Keeley J, Mayer T G, Cox R 1986 Quantification of lumbar function: Part 5. Reliability of range of motion measures in the sagittal plane and in an in vivo torso rotation technique. Spine 11: 31–35

Kelsey J L, Munat D J, Golden A L 1992 Epidemiology of low back pain. In: Jayson M I V (ed) The lumbar spine and back pain. Churchill Livingstone, Edinburgh

Kemmer F W, Bisping R, Steingruber H J, Baar H, Hardtmann F, Schlaghecke R, Berger M

1986 Psychological stress and metabolic control in patients with diabetes mellitus. New England Journal of Medicine 314: 1078–1084

Kenshalo D R Jr, Willis W D Jr 1991 The role of the cerebral cortex in pain sensation. In: Peters A (ed) Cerebral cortex. Plenum Press, New York, vol 9, pp 153–212

Kerr F W L 1975 Neuroanatomical substrates of nociception in the spinal cord. Pain 1: 325

Kinney R K, Gatchel R J, Mayer T G 1991 The SCL-90R evaluated as an alternative to the MMPI for psychological screening of chronic low back pain patients. Spine 16: 940–942

Kirkaldy-Willis W H 1988 Managing low back pain. Churchill Livingstone, Edinburgh

Kitchen S, Bazin S 1996 Clayton's electrotherapy, 10th ed. WB Saunders, London

Klaber-Moffett J A, Richardson P H 1995 The influence of psychological variables on the development and perception of musculoskeletal pain. Physiotherapy Theory and Practice 11: 3–11

Klaber-Moffett J, Richardson G, Sheldon T A, Maynard A 1995 Back pain. Its management and cost to society. University of York, York

Klaber-Moffett J A, Chase S M, Portek I, Ennis J R 1986 A controlled prospective trial to evaluate the effectiveness of a back school in the relief of chronic low back pain. Spine 11: 120–22

Klapow J C, Slater M A, Patterson T L, Doctor J N, Atkinson J H, Garfin S R 1993 An empirical evaluation of multidimensional clinical outcome in chronic low back pain patients. Pain 55: 107–118

Klein A B, Synder-Mackler L, Roy S H, Deluca C J 1991 Comparison of spinal mobility and isometric trunk extensor forces with electromyographic spectral analysis in identifying low back pain. Physical Therapy 71: 445–454

Koes B W, Bouter L M, Beckerman H, van der Heijden G J M G, Knipschild P G 1991 Physiotherapy exercises and back pain: a blinded review. British Medical Journal 302: 1572

Korsch B M, Negrete V F 1972 Doctor–patient communication. Scientific American 227: 66–74

Korsch B M, Gozzi E K, Francis V 1968 Gaps in doctor–patient communication. Paediatrics 42: 855–871

Kravitz E, Moore M E, Glaros A 1981 Paralumbar muscle activity in chronic low back pain. Archives of Physical Medicine and Rehabilitation 62: 172–176

Kreitman E, Sainsbury P 1965 Hypochondriasis in out-patients at a general hospital. British Journal of Psychiatry 111: 607–615

Krishnan K R R, France R D, Pelton S, McCann U D, Davidson J, Urban B J 1985 Chronic pain and depression II. Symptoms of anxiety in chronic low back pain patients and their relationship to subtypes of depression. Pain 22: 289–294

Kruger L, Liebeskind J C (eds) Advances in pain research and therapy. Raven Press, New York, vol VI

LaCroix J M, Clarke M A, Bock J C, Doxey N, Wood A, Lavis S 1983 Biofeedback and relaxation in the treatment of migraine headaches: comparative effectiveness and physiological correlates. Journal of Neurology, Neurosurgery and Psychiatry 46: 525–532

Lamb J F, Ingram C G, Johnston I A, Pitman R M 1980 Introduction to physiology. Blackwell Scientific Publications, Oxford

Lamour Y, Willer J C, Guilbaud G 1982 Neuronal responses to noxious stimulation in the rat somatosensory cortex. Neuroscience Letters 29: 35

Lang P J, Kozak M J, Miller G A, Levin D N, McLean A 1980 Emotional imagery: conceptual structure and pattern of somato-visceral response. Psychophysiology 17: 179–192

Lankhurst G J, van de Stadt R J, Vogelaar T W, van der Korst J K, Prevo A J H 1982 Objectivity and repeatability of measurement in low back pain. Scandinavian Journal of Rehabilitation Medicine 14: 21–26

Lasagna L 1960 The clinical measurement of pain. Annals of the New York Academy of Sciences 86: 28–37

Le Blanc H J, Gatipon G B 1974 Medial bulboreticular responses to peripherally applied noxious stimuli. Experimental Neurology 42: 264

Leavitt F, Garron L 1980 Validity of a back pain classification scale for detecting psychological disturbance as measured by the MMPI. Journal of Clinical Psychology 36: 186–189

LeBoeuf A 1980 Effects of frontalis biofeedback on subjective ratings of relaxation. Perceptual and Motor Skills 50: 99–103

Lethem J, Slade P D, Troup J D G, Bentley G 1983 The fear avoidance model of exaggerated pain perception. Behaviour Research and Therapy 21: 401–408

Lewis V A et al 1971 Evaluation of the periaqueductal central grey (PAG) as a morphine specific locus of action and examination of morphine induced stimulation produced analgesia coincident at PAG loci. Brain Research 124: 283

Ley P 1972 Primacy, rated importance and recall of medical information. Journal of Health and Social Behavior 13: 311–317

Ley P, Spelman M S 1965 Communication in an out patient setting. British Journal of Sociology and Clinical Psychology 4: 114

Ley P, Spelman M S 1967 Communicating with the patient. Staples Press, London

Ley P, Bradshaw D, Eaves D, Walker C M A 1973 A method for increasing patients recall of information presented by doctors. Psychological Medicine 3: 217

Light A R, Perl E R 1979 Re-examination of the dorsal root projection to the spinal dorsal horn including observations in the differential termination of coarse and fine fibres. Journal of Comparative Neurology 186: 117

Lindsley D B 1970 The role of non specific reticulothalamocortical systems in emotion. In: Black P (ed) Physiological correlates of emotion. Academic Press, New York

Linton S J 1994 The challenge of preventing chronic musculoskeletal pain. Proceedings of the 7th World Congress on Pain. In: Gebhart G F, Hammond D L, Jensen T S (eds) Progress in pain research and management. IASP Press, Seattle

Linton S J, Gotestam K G 1985 Controlling pain reports through operant conditioning: a laboratory demonstration. Perceptual and Motor Skills 60: 427–437

Lipton S 1979 The control of chronic pain. Edward Arnold, London

Lopez Ibor J J 1972 Masked depressions. British Journal of Psychiatry 120: 245–258

Lowe P V 1970 The art of communication. Physiotherapy 56: 182–187

Luiselli J K, Marholin D, Steinman D L, Steinman W M 1979 Assessing the effects of relaxation training. Behavior Therapy 10: 663–668

Luthe W (ed) 1969 Autogenic therapy. Grune & Stratton, New York, vols 1–6

Lyles J N, Burish T G, Krozely M G, Oldham R K 1982 Efficacy of relaxation training and guided imagery in reducing the aversiveness of cancer chemotherapy. Journal of Consulting and Clinical Psychology 50: 509–524

Maas J W 1972 Adrenocortical steroid hormones, electrolytes and the disposition of the catecholamines with particular reference to depressive states. Journal of Psychiatric Research 9: 227–241

McCain G A, Scudds R A 1988 The concept of primary fibromyalgia (fibrositis): clinical value, relation and significance to other chronic musculoskeletal pain syndromes. Pain 33: 273

McCreary C, Turner J, Dawson E 1979 The MMPI as a predictor of response to conservative treatment of low back pain. Journal of Clinical Psychology 35: 278–284

McCreary C, Turner J, Dawson E 1980 Emotional disturbance and chronic low back pain. Journal of Clinical Psychology 36: 709–715

McDaniel J 1971 Metabolic and CNS correlates of cognitive dysfuction with renal failure. Psychophysiology 8: 704–713

MacEvilly M, Buggy D 1996 Back pain and pregnancy: a review. Pain 64: 405–414

McGrady A V, Yonker R, Tan S Y, Fine T H, Woerner M 1981 The effects of biofeedback-assisted relaxation training on blood pressure and selected biochemical parameters in patients with essential hypertension. Biofeedback and Self-Regulation 6: 343–353

McGuigan F J 1984 Progressive relaxation, origins, principles, and clinical applications. In: Woolfolk R L, Lehrer P M (eds) Principles and practice of stress management. Guilford Press, New York

McIntosh J 1974 Process of communication, information seeking and control associated with cancer. Social Science and Medicine 8: 167–187

McNeill T, Warwick D, Anserrsson G, Schultz A 1980 Trunk strengths in attempted flexion, extension and lateral bending in healthy subjects and patients with low back disorders. Spine 5: 529–538

Magora A 1975 Investigation of the relationship between LBP and occupation. VII Neurology and orthopaedic conditions. Scandinavian Journal of Rehabilitation Medicine 7: 6–151

Maguire P 1985 Barriers to psychological care of the dying. British Medical Journal 291: 1711–1713

Main C J 1983 The modified somatic perception questionnaire. Journal of Psychosomatic Research 27: 503–514

Main C J 1992 Psychological assessment of pain. Paper presented at 23rd Annual Meeting of AAPB, Colorado Springs

Main C J 1992 Psychological treatment. In: Jayson M I V (ed) The lumbar spine and back pain. Churchill Livingstone, Edinburgh

Main C J, Waddell G 1984 The detection of psychological abnormality in chronic low back pain using four simple scales. Current Concepts in Pain 2: 10–15

Main C J, Waddell G 1987 Personality assessment in the management of low back pain. Clinical Rehabilitation 1: 139–142

Main C J, Evans P J D, Whitehead R C 1991 An investigation of personality structure and other psychological features in patients presenting with low back pain: a critique of the MMPI. In: Bond M R, Charlton J E, Woolf C J (eds) Proceedings of VIth World Congress of Pain, Elsevier Science Publishers, Amsterdam

Main C J, Wood P L R, Hollis S, Spoanswick C C, Waddell G 1992 The distress and risk assessment method: a simple classification to identify distress and evaluate the risk of poor outcome. Spine 17: 42–52

Mancia M, Otero-Costas J 1973 Nature of midbrain influences upon thalamic neurons. Brain Research 49: 200

Marbach J J, Richlin D M, Lipton J A 1983 Illness behaviour, depression and anhedonia in myofascial face and back pain patients. Psychotherapy and Psychosomatics 39: 47–54

Mason J W 1971 A re-evaluation of the concept of non-specificity in stress theory. Journal of Psychiatric Research 8: 323–333

Mathew R J, Ho B T Kralik, P, Taylor D, Semchuk K, Weinman M, Claghorn J L 1980 Catechol-o-methyltransferase and catecholamines in anxiety and relaxation. Psychiatric Research 3: 85–91

Mathews J J 1983 The communication process in clinical settings. Social Science and Medicine 17: 1371–1378

Maule A G, Shaw C, Halton D W, Johnston C F, Fairweather I, Buchanan K D 1989 Tachykinin immunoreactivity in the parasitic flatworm *diclidophora merlangi* and its fish host the whiting *merlangius merlangus*: radioimmunoassay and chromatographic characterisation using region specific substance P and neurokinin A antisera. Comprehensive Biochemical Physiology 94C: 533–541

Mayer D J, Hayes R L 1975 Stimulation produced analgesia. Development of tolerance and cross tolerance to morphine. Science 188: 941

Mayer D J, Liebeskind J C 1974 Pain reduction by focal electrical stimulation of the brain: anatomical and behavioural analysis. Brain Research 68: 77

Mayer T G, Tencer A F, Kristofferson J, Mooney V 1984 Use of non invasive techniques for quantification of spinal range of motion in normal subjects and chronic low back dysfunction patients. Spine 9: 588–595

Mayou R 1991 Medically unexplained physical symptoms. British Medical Journal 30: 534

Meade T W, Dyer S, Browne W, Townsend J, Frank A O 1990 Low back pain of mechanical origin: randomised comparison of chiropractic and hospital out-patient treatment. British Medical Journal 300: 1431–1437

Meade W, Chakrabarti R, Haines A P, North W R S, Stirling Y 1979 Characteristics affecting fibrinolytic activity and plasma fibrinogen concentrations. British Medical Journal 1: 153–156

Mechanic D 1962 The concept of illness behaviour. Journal of Chronic Diseases 15: 189–194

Mechanic D 1978 Medical sociology. Collier Macmillan, London

Mellin G 1985 Physical therapy for chronic low back pain: correlations between spinal mobility and treatment outcome. Scandinavian Journal of Rehabilitation Medicine 17: 163–166

Mellin G 1987 Method and instrument for non invasive measurements of thoracolumbar rotation. Spine 12: 28–31

Melzack R 1981 Myofascial trigger points: relation to acupuncture and mechanisms of pain. Archives of Physical Medicine and Rehabilitation 62: 114–117

Melzack R, Wall P D 1965 Pain mechanisms. A new theory. Science 150: 971–979

Melzack R, Wall P D 1988 The challenge of pain. Penguin, Harmondsworth

Melzack R, Wall P 1989 Textbook of pain. Churchill Livingstone, Edinburgh

Merskey H 1965 Psychiatric patients with persistent pain. Journal of Psychosomatic Research 9: 299–309

Merskey H, Spear F G 1967 Pain. Psychological and psychiatric aspects. Baillière Tindall, London

Messing R B, Lyttle L D 1977 Serotonin containing neurons: their possible role in pain and analgesia. Pain 4: 1

Michaels R R, Parra J, McCann D S, Vander A J 1979 Renin, cortisol, and aldosterone during transcendental meditation. Psychosomatic Medicine 41: 50–54

Middaugh S J, Kee W G 1987 Advances in EMG monitoring and biofeedback in the treatment of chronic cervical and low back pain. Advances in Clinical Rehabilitation 1: 137–172

Miller C, Cooper P J 1988 Adult abnormal psychology. Churchill Livingstone, Edinburgh

Montagu A 1978 Touching and the human significance of the skin. Harper & Row, New York

Morrell P M, Hollandsworth J G 1986 Norepinephrine alterations under stress conditions following the regular practice of meditation. Psychosomatic Medicine 48: 270–277

Morrison D C, Henson P M 1978 Release of mediators from mast cells and basophils induced by different stimuli. In: Bach M K (ed) Immediate hypersensitivity: modern concepts and developments. Marcel Dekker, New York, pp 431–502

Murase K, Randic M 1984 Actions of substance P on rat spinal dorsal horn neurons. Journal of Physiology 436: 203

Murray J B 1982 Psychological aspects of low back pain. Psychological Reports 50: 343–351

Narita T, Satoshi M, Yagi T 1987 Psychophysiological analysis during autogenic training. Advances in Biological Psychiatry 16: 72–89

Nathan P W 1976 The gate-control theory of pain—a critical review. Brain 99: 123–158

Nawa H, Hirose T, Takashima H, Inayama S, Nakanishi S 1983 Nucleotide sequence of cloned cDNA's for two types of bovine brain substance P precursor. Nature 306:

Nicholas M K, Wilson P H, Goyen J 1992 A comparison of cognitive–behavioural group treatment and an alternative non psychological treatment for chronic low back pain. Pain 48: 339–347

Nigl A J, Fischer-Williams M 1980 Treatment of low back strain with electromyographic biofeedback and relaxation training. Psychosomatics 21: 495–499

Nouwen A, Bush C 1984 Relationship between paraspinal EMG and chronic LBP. Pain 20: 109–123

Nouwen A, Solinger J W 1979 The effectiveness of EMG biofeedback training in low back pain. Biofeedback and Self Regulation 4: 103–111

Nouwen A, Van Akkerveeken P F, Versloot J M 1987 Patterns of muscular activity during movement in patients with chronic low back pain. Spine 12: 777–782

Nuki G 1983 Non steroidal analgesic and antiinflammatory agents. British Medical Journal 289: 39–43

Ohnhaus E E, Adler R 1975 Methodological problems in the measurement of pain: a comparison between the verbal rating scale and the visual analogue scale. Pain 1: 379–384

Orne M T 1992 Nonpharmacological approaches to pain relief: hypnosis, biofeedback, placebo effects. In: Aronoff G M (ed) Evaluation and treatment of chronic pain. Williams & Wilkins, Baltimore, pp 430–439

Osterweis M, Kleinman A, Mechanic D 1987 Pain and disability. National Academy Press, Washington

Otsuka M, Takahashi T 1979 Putative peptide neurotransmitters. Annual Review of Pharmacology and Toxicology 17: 425–439

Park L C, Covi L 1965 Non blind placebo trial: an experiment of neurotic patients response to placebo when its inert content is disclosed. Archives of General Psychiatry 12: 336–345

Parris W E V, Kambam J R, Naukam R J, Rama Sastry B V 1990 Immunoreactive substance P is decreased in the saliva of patients with chronic back pain syndromes. Anesthesia and Analgesia 70: 63–7

Patel C 1984 Yogic therapy. In: Woolfolk R L, Lehrer P M (eds) Principles and practice of stress management. Guilford Press, New York

Payton O D 1983 Effects of instruction in basic communication skills on physical therapist and physical therapy students. Physical Therapy 63: 1292–1297

Pearcey M 1986 Measurement of spinal mobility. Clinical Biomechanics 1: 44–51

Peck C 1982 Controlling chronic pain. Fontana, London

Peck C, Kraft G 1977 Electromyographic biofeedback for pain related to muscle tension. Archives of Surgery 112: 889–895

Pendleton D A, Bochner S 1980 The communication of medical information in general practice consultations as a function of patients social class. Social Science and Medicine 14: 669–673

Pendleton D, Schofield T, Tate P, Havelock P 1984 The consultation: an approach to learning and teaching. Oxford University Press, Oxford

Penfield W 1975 The mystery of the mind. Princeton University Press, New Jersey

Perl G S, Anderson K V 1978 Response pattern of cells in the feline caudal nucleus reticularis gigantocellularis after noxious trigeminal and spinal stimulation. Experimental Neurology 58: 271

Perl G S, Anderson K V 1980 Interactions between nucleus centrum medianum and gigantocellularis nociceptive neurons. Brain Research Bulletin 5: 203

Pickering T G, James G D, Boddie C, Harshfield G A, Blank S, Laragh J H 1988 How common is white coat hypertension? Journal of the American Medical Association 259: 225–228

Pilowsky I 1970 Primary and secondary hypochondriasis. Acta Psychiatrica Scandinavica 46: 273–285

Pilowsky I, Spence N D 1975a Illness behaviour syndromes associated with intractable pain. Pain 2: 61–71

Pilowsky I, Spence N D 1975b Patterns of illness behaviour in patients with intractable pain. Journal of Psychosomatic Research 19: 279–287

Pilowsky I, Spence N D 1976 Is illness behaviour related to chronicity in patients with intractable pain. Pain 2: 61–71

Polatin P B, Mayer T G 1992 Quantification of function in chronic low back pain. In: Turk D C, Melzack R (eds) Handbook of pain assessment. Guilford Press, New York

Polatin P B, Kinney R K, Gatchel R J, Lillo E, Mayer T G 1993 Psychiatric illness and chronic low back pain. The mind and the spine-which goes first? Spine 18: 66–71

Poulton E C 1977 Qualitative subjective assessments are almost always biased, sometimes completely misleading. British Journal of Psychology 68: 409–411

Prokop C K, Bradley L 1980 Mutivariate analysis of the MMPI profiles of patients with multiple pain complaints. Journal of Personality Assessment 44: 246–252

Quint J C 1965 Institutionalised practices of information control. Psychiatry 28: 119–132

Raab W 1968 Correlated cardiovascular, adrenergic and adrenocortical responses to sensory and mental annoyances in man. a potential accessory cardiac risk factor. Psychosomatic Medicine 30: 809–818

Rachman S L, Philips C 1978 Psychology and medicine. Penguin, Harmondsworth

Rang H P, Dale M M 1991 Pharmacology, 2nd edn. Churchill Livingstone, Edinburgh

Recht L D, Abrams G M 1986 Neuropeptides and their role in nociception and analgesia. Neurology Clinics 4: 833–852

Redd W H, Porterfield A L, Anderson B L 1979 Behavior modification: behavioral approaches to human problems. Random House, New York

Reis D J 1988 The brain and hypertension. Archives of Neurology 45: 180–183

Reynolds P M G 1975 Measurement of spinal mobility: a comparison of three methods. Rheumatology and Rehabilitation 14: 180

Riddoch J, Lennon S 1991 Evaluation of practice. Physiotherapy 77: 439–444

Rimon A, Le Greves P, Nyberg F, Heikkela L, Salmela L, Terenius L 1984 Elevation of substance P like immunoreactivity in the CSF of psychiatric patients. Biological Psychiatry 19: 509–516

Robbins S L, Angell M, Kumar V 1981 Basic pathology, 3rd edn. W B Saunders, London

Rogers H J, Spector R G, Trounce J R 1985 Textbook of clinical pharmacology. Hodder & Stoughton, London

Roland M, Morris R 1983 A study of the natural history of low back pain. Spine 8: 141–144

Romano J A, Turner J A 1985 Chronic pain and depression: does the evidence support a relationship. Psychological Bulletin 97: 18–34

Rose M J, Klenerman L, Atchison L, Slade P D 1992 A comparison of three chronic pain conditions using the fear avoidance model of exaggerated pain perception. Behaviour Research and Therapy 30: 359–365

Rose M J, Slade P D, Reilly J P, Dewey M 1995 A comparative analysis of psychological and physical models of low back pain experience. Physiotherapy 81: 710–716

Rosenthal A K, Keefe F J 1983 The use of coping strategies in chronic low back pain patients: relationship of patient characteristics and current adjustment. Pain 17: 33–34

Roth J A 1963 Information and the control of treatment in tuberculosis hospitals. In: Friedson E (ed) Hospitals in modern society. Free Press, New York

Roy S H, DeLuca C J, Snyder-Mackler L 1990 Fatigue, recovery and low back pain in elite rowers. Medicine and Science in Sports and Exercise 22: 463–469

Ruda M A, Bennett C J, Dubner R 1986 Neurochemistry and neurocircuitry in the dorsal horn. Progress in Brain Research 66: 219

Rudy T E, Kerns R D, Turk D C 1988 Chronic pain and depression: toward a cognitive–behavioural model. Pain 35: 129–140

Sainsbury P 1960 Neuroticism in unselected out-patients attending physical medicine plus orthopaedic departments. Annals of Physical Medicine 5: 310–317

Sainsbury P, Gibson J G 1954 Symptoms of anxiety and tension and accompanying physiological changes in the muscular system. Journal of Neurology, Neurosurgery and Psychiatry 17: 216

Schneider C J 1987 Cost effectiveness of biofeedback and behavioral medicine treatments: a review of the literature. Biofeedback and Self Regulation 12: 71–92

Schneider C, Wilson E 1985 Foundations of biofeedback practice. Biofeedback Society of America, Colorado

Schultz J H, Luthe W 1969 Autogenic therapy vol. I: autogenic methods. Grune & Stratton, New York

Schuster M M 1983 Biofeedback control of gastrointestinal motility. In: Basmajian J V (ed) Biofeedback. Principles and practice for clinicians. Williams & Wilkins, Baltimore

Schwartz M S 1987 Biofeedback. A practitioners guide. Guilford Press, New York

Schwartz T 1978 Physiological psychology, 2nd edn. Prentice Hall, London

Seligman M E 1968 Chronic fear produced by unpredictable electric shock. Journal of Comparative and Physiological Psychology 66: 402–411

Seligman M E P 1975 Helplessness: on depression, development and death. Freeman, San Francisco

Selkurt E 1975 Basic physiology for the health sciences. Little Brown, Boston

Selye H 1978 The stress of life. McGraw Hill, New York

Shanfield S B, Killingsworth R N 1977 Psychiatric aspects of pain. Annals of Psychiatry 7: 24–35

Shedivy D I, Kleinman K M 1977 Lack of correlation between frontalis EMG and either neck EMG or verbal ratings of tension. Psychophysiology 14: 182–186

Sherman R, Goeken A, DeGood D, Glaros A, Blanchard E, Andrasik F, Wolf S, Arena J 1995 March biofeedback for pain: a multipractitioner outcome study. Paper presented at the 26th annual convention of the Association for Applied Psychophysiology and Biofeedback, Cincinnati, Ohio

Sim J 1989 Truthfulness in the therapeutic relationship. Physiotherapy Practice 5: 121–122

Simpson M E 1980 Societal support and education. In: Kutask I W, Schlesinger L B (eds) Handbook on stress and anxiety. Jossey-Bass, San Francisco

Smik R 1973 Frontalis muscle tension and personality. Psychophysiology 10: 311–312

Snook S H 1982 Low back pain in industry. In: White A A, Gordon S L (eds) American Academy of Orthopaedic Surgeons symposium on idiopathic low back pain. CV Mosby, St Louis, pp 23–38

Sokolov N E 1963 Perception and the coordinated reflex. Pergamon, New York

Spence N D 1984 Relaxation training for chronic pain patients using EMG feedback: an analysis of process and outcome effects. Australian and New Zealand Journal of Psychiatry 18: 263–272

Spengler S 1980 Personality characteristics and pain. In: Elton D (ed) Psychological control of pain. Grune & Stratton, Australia

Spiro H M 1986 Doctors, patients and placebos. Yale University Press, London

Spitzer W O 1987 Scientific approach to the assessment and management of activity related spinal disorders. A monograph for clinicians. Report of the Quebec Task Force on Spinal Disorders. Spine 12 (suppl 1): 1–59

Stankovic R, Johnell O 1990 Conservative treatment of acute low back pain: a prospective randomized trial. Spine 15: 120–123

Stein J F 1982 Introduction to neurophysiology. Blackwell Scientific Publications, Oxford

Sternbach R 1986 The psychology of pain. Raven Press, New York

Stimson G V 1974 Obeying doctors orders: a view from the other side. Social Science and Medicine 8: 97

Strecher V J 1984 Improving physician–patient interaction: a review. Patient Counselling and Health Education 4: 129

Strongman K 1987 The psychology of emotion. John Wiley, Chichester

Swanson D W 1984 Chronic pain as a third pathologic emotion. American Journal of Psychiatry 141: 210–214

Szentagothai J 1964 neuronal and synaptic arrangements in the substantia gelatinosa rolandi. Journal of Comprehensive Neurology 122: 219

Talbot J D, Marrett S, Evans A C, Meyer E, Bushnell M C, Duncan G H 1991 Multiple representations of pain in human cerebral cortex. Science 251: 1355–1358

Taub E, Stroebel C 1978 Biofeedback in the treatment of vasoconstrictive syndromes. Biofeedback and Self Regulation 3: 363–374

Taylor D N, Lee C T 1991 Lack of correlation between frontalis electromyography and self-ratings of either frontalis tension or state anxiety. Perceptual and Motor Skills 72: 1131–1134

Taylor W 1990 EMG biofeedback in the assessment and treatment of myofascial pain syndromes. Paper presented at 21st Annual Meeting of the Association of Applied Psychophysiology and Biofeedback, Washington, DC

Tollison C D 1989 Handbook of clinical pain management. Williams & Wilkins, Baltimore

Torebjork H E, Hallin R G 1973 Perceptual changes accompanying controlled preferential blocking of A and C fibre responses in intact human nerves. Experimental Brain Research 16: 321

Travell J, Simons D 1983 Myofascial pain and dysfunction: the trigger point manual. Williams & Wilkins, Baltimore

Tucker D M 1981 Lateral brain function, emotion and conceptualisation. Psychological Bulletin 89: 19–46

Turk D C, Flor H 1983 Etiological theories and treatment for chronic back pain II. Psycholgical models-interventions. Pain 19: 209–233

Turk D C, Flor H, Rudy T E 1987 Pain and families I. Etiology, maintenance and psychosocial impact. Pain 30: 3–27

Turk D C, Rudy T E 1991 Neglected topics in the treatment of chronic pain patients: relapses, non compliance and adherence enhancement. Pain 44: 5–28

Turk D C, Melzack R 1992 Handbook of pain assessment. Guilford Press, New York

Turk D C, Meichenbaum D, Genest M 1983 Pain and behavioral medicine. Guilford Press, New York

Turner J A, Chapman C R 1982 Psychological intervention for chronic pain: a critical review I. Relaxation training and biofeedback. Pain 12: 1–21

Turner J A, Romano J M 1990 Cognitive–behavioral therapy. In: Bonica J J (ed) Management of pain. Lea & Febiger, Philadelphia, pp 1711–1721

Ullman L P, Krasner L 1975 A psychological approach to abnormal behaviour. Prentice Hall, New Jersey

Ursin H, Baade E, Levine S 1978 Psychobiology of stress: a study of coping man. Academic Press, New York

Vallfors B 1985 Acute, subacute and chronic low back pain: clinical symptoms, absenteeism and working environment. Scandinavian Journal of Rehabilitation Medicine, Supplement 11: 1–98

Van Hees J, Gybels J 1981 C nociceptive activity in human nerve during painful and non-painful skin stimulation. Journal of Neurology, Neurosurgery and Psychiatry 44: 600

Von Euler U S, Gaddum J H 1931 An unidentified depressor substance in certain tissue extracts. Journal Physiology London 72: 74–87

Vukmir R D 1991 Low back pain. Review of diagnosis and treatment. American Journal of Emergency Medicine 9: 328–335

Waddell G 1987 A new clinical model for the treatment of low back pain. 1987 Volvo Award in Clinical Sciences. Spine 12: 632–644

Waddell G 1987 Clinical assessment of lumbar impairment. Clinical Orthopaedics 221: 110–120

Waddell G, Turk D C 1992 Clinical assessment of low back pain. In: Turk D C, Melzack R (eds) Handbook of pain assessment. Guilford Press, New York

Waddell G, Main C J, Morris E W, Venner R M, Rae P S, Sharmy S H, Galloway H 1982 Normality and reliability in the clinical assessment of backache. British Medical Journal 284: 1519

Waddell G, McCulloch J A, Kummel E, Veenner R M 1980 Non-organic physical signs in low back pain. Spine 5: 117–125

Waddell G, Bircher M, Finlayson D, Main C J 1984 Symptoms and signs. Physical disease or illness behaviour? British Medical Journal 289: 740

Waddell G, Main C J, Morris E W, DiPaola M, Gray I C M 1984 Chronic low back pain, psychological distress and illness behaviour. Spine 9: 209–213

Wagstaff G F 1982 A small dose of commonsense–communication, persuasion and physiotherapy. Physiotherapy 68: 327–329

Waitzkin H, Stoeckle J D 1972 The communication of information about illness. Advances in Psychosomatic Medicine 8: 180–215

Walker A E, Thompson A F, McQueen J D 1953 Behaviour and the temporal rhinencephalon in the monkey. Bulletin of the Johns Hopkins Hospital 93: 63–92

Walsh D 1991 Ascending nociceptive pathways: relevance to the physiotherapist. Physiotherapy 77: 317–321

Walsh K, Varnes N, Osmond C, Styles R, Coggon D 1989 Occupational causes of low back pain. Scandinavian Journal of Work, Environment and Health 15: 54–59

Walsh T D 1983 Antidepressants in chronic pain. Clinical Neuropharmacology 6: 271

Ward N, Bloom V 1982 Psychobiological markers in coexisting pain and depression: toward a unified theory. Journal of Clinical Psychiatry 43: 32–39

Weisenberg M 1977 Pain and pain control. Psychological Bulletin 84: 1008–1044

Weisenberg M 1989 Cognitive aspects of pain. In: Melzack R, Wall P D (eds) Textbook of pain. Churchill Livingstone, Edinburgh

Wells P, Frampton V, Bowsher D 1988 Pain management and control in physiotherapy. Heinemann Physiotherapy, London

Wickramasekera I 1987 Biofeedback and behaviour modification for chronic pain. In: Echternach J L (ed) Pain. Clinics in physical therapy. Churchill Livingstone, New York, vol XII

Wile D 1985 Cheng Man-Ching's advanced t'ai-chi form instructions. Sweet Ch'i Press, New York

Wilkinson H A 1983 Failed back syndrome. Etiology and therapy. Harper & Row, London

Willer J C, Albe-Fessard D 1983 Further studies on the role of afferent input from relatively large diameter fibres in transmission of nociceptive messages in humans. Brain Research 278: 318

Willer J C, Boureau F, Albe-Fessard D 1978 Role of large diameter cutaneous afferents in transmission of nociceptive messages: electrophysiological study in man. Brain Research 152: 358

Williams J I 1989 Illness behaviour to wellness behaviour. The ' school for bravery' approach. Physiotherapy 75: 2–7

Williams P, Warwick R 1980 Gray's anatomy, 36th edn. Churchill Livingstone, Edinburgh

Willis W D 1984 Modulation of primate spinothalamic tract discharges. In: Kruger L, Liebeskind J C (eds) Advances in pain research and therapy. Raven Press, New York, vol VI

Willson P, McNamara J R 1982 How perceptions of a simulated physician–patient interaction influence intended satisfaction and compliance. Social Science and Medicine 16: 1699–1704

Wilson E 1990 Interactive EEG biofeedback. Paper presented at the 21st Annual Meeting of the AAPB, Washington, DC

Winkelman R K 1968 Kinins from human skin. In: Kenshalo D R (ed) The skin senses. Springfield, New York, pp 499–511

Wolf S L 1983 Neurophysiological factors in electromyographic feedback for neuromotor disturbances. In: Basmajian J V (ed) Biofeedback principles and practice for clinicians. Williams & Wilkins, Baltimore, pp 5–22

Wolf S L, Rao V 1982 Transcutaneous electrical stimulation. Use and abuse. In: Brens S F, Chapman S L (eds) Management of patients with chronic pain. MTP Press, Boston

Wolf S L, Wolf L B, Segal R L 1989 The relationship of extraneous movements to lumbar paraspinal muscle activity: implications for EMG biofeedback training applications to low back pain patients. Biofeedback and Self Regulation 14: 63–74

Wolfer J A, Davies C 1970 Assessment of surgical patients pre-operative emotional condition and post operative welfare. Nursing Research 19: 402–414

Wolff H G 1963 Headache and other head pain. Oxford University Press, New York

Wolkind S N 1974 Psychiatric aspects of low back pain. Physiotherapy 60: 75–77

Wolman B B 1965 Handbook of clinical psychology. McGraw Hill, New York

Wolpe J 1973 The practice of behavior therapy (2nd edn). Pergamon Press, New York

Woodforde J M, Merskey H 1972 Personality traits of patients with chronic pain. Journal of Psychosomatic Research 16: 1

Wu W H, Smith L G 1987 Pain management. Assessment of acute and chronic syndromes. Human Sciences Press, New York

Wyke B 1987 Neurological aspects of low back pain. In: Jayson M I V (ed) The lumbar spine and back pain. Pitman Medical, Kent

Wyke B D 1981 Neurological aspects of pain therapy. In: Swerdlow M (ed) The therapy of pain, 1st edn. MTP Press, Lancaster

Yaksh T L 1986 The central pharmacology of primary afferents with emphasis on the disposition and role of primary afferent substance P. In: Yaksh T L (ed) Spinal afferent processing. Plenum Press, New York

Yaksh T L, Aimone L D 1990 The central pharmacology of pain transmission. In: Bonica J J (ed) Management of pain. Lea & Febiger, Philadelphia, vol I

Yaksh T L, Hammond D L 1982 Peripheral and central substrates in the rostral transmission of nociceptive information. Pain 13: 1

Yaksh T L, Rudy T A 1978 Narcotic analgesics: CNS sites and mechanisms of action as revealed by intracerebral injection techniques. Pain 4: 299

Zborowski M 1952 Cultural components in responses to pain. Journal of Social Issues 8: 16–30

Zborowski M 1969 People in pain. Jossey-Bass, San Francisco

Zhuo D, Dighe J, Basmajian J V 1983 EMG biofeedback and Chinese 'Chi Kung' relaxation effects in patients with low back pain. Physiotherapy 35: 13–18

Zimbardo P, Ebbeson E, Maslach C 1977 Influencing attitudes and changing behaviour. Addison Wesley, Massachusetts

Zola I K 1966 Culture and symptoms: an analysis of patients presenting complaints. American Sociological Review 31: 615–638

Zung W W K 1965 A self-rating depression scale. Archives of General Psychiatry 32: 63–70

Glossary

Alexithymia. Literally means without words for feelings. It is a finding in psychosomatic and addictive disorders where emotions are poorly differentiated and the person tends to express their emotions as somatic symptoms.

Allodynia. A neurophysiologically and neurochemically mediated phenomenon whereby a number of sensory terminals around an area of tissue damage become hypersensitive responding to non-noxious stimuli with a pain response pattern.

Amygdala. An area of the cerebral cortex that is involved in emotional states.

Antidepressant. A drug that relieves depression.

Anxiety. A personality characteristic of responding to certain situations with a stress syndrome of responses. Trait anxiety is a characteristic of the individual and state anxiety is associated with a particular situation.

Arousal. A general level of activation that is reflected in several physiological systems and can be measured by electrical activity in e.g. brain, heart rate, muscle activity, etc.

Autogenic training. A system of psychosomatic self-regulation designed to support the central mechanisms responsible for homeostatic processes. The system is designed to facilitate a shift towards relaxation in different somatic systems such as the neuromuscular and vascular systems.

Autonomic nervous system. A subsystem of the peripheral nervous system that carries messages between the CNS and the heart, lungs and other organs and glands in the body. The ANS regulates the activity of these organs and glands to meet varying demands placed upon the body and also provides information to the brain about that activity.

Behavioural model. This model defines pain by the presence of pain behaviours which are verbal and nonverbal signs of distress that are independent of subjective report. Using this model, pain becomes chronic because the pain behaviour is positively reinforced while well behaviour is not reinforced.

Biofeedback. Biofeedback is a self-regulation training strategy where a patient is attached to physiological monitoring equipment via surface sensors. These sensors relay information about the internal physiological environment which was not previously discriminated by the individual to machines which measure and display it audibly and visually making the information available for use in learning to create change in a desired direction.

Central nervous system. The brain and spinal cord. Primary function is to process information provided by the sensory systems and decide upon an appropriate action for the motor system.

Cerebellum. The part of the brain at the back of the skull. Function is to control finely co-ordinated movements.

Cerebral cortex. Outer surface of the cerebrum, consisting of two cerebral hemisheres. It is anatomically divided into four areas, the frontal, parietal, occipital and temporal lobe. It is divided functionally into the sensory cortex, motor cortex and association cortex.

Cerebrum (also referred to as the telencephalon). This is the largest part of the forebrain. It is divided into the right and left cerebral hemispheres and contains the striatum and the limbic system.

Circadian rhythm. A repeating cycle such as waking or sleeping.

Cognitive model. This model examines constructs such as expectations and beliefs about pain, personal control, problem-solving abilities and coping skills. The model addresses these cognitive processes and suggests that emotional distress or behavioural difficulty is not a direct reaction to an untoward life event, but rather a direct consequence of how that event is perceived.

Cognitive-behavioural model. A unifying theory in which the behavioural model is expanded to incorporate cognition and affect within behaviour therapy. A variety of psychological interventions are combined within this framework and it emphasises education, control by the patient and coping strategies.

Cognitive restructuring. A therapy technique or process for coping with stress or pain that involves replacing stress or pain provoking thoughts with more constructive thoughts in order to make the experience less threatening and disruptive.

Conversion disorder. A somatoform disorder where a mental conflict is translated into a physical disorder.

Depression. An excessively sad mood without obvious cause or disproportional to the problem.

Dysthymia. A pattern of depression in which the person shows sad mood, lack of interest and loss of pleasure. Associated with major depressive disorder but to a lesser degree.

Empathy. The way in which a person attempts to appreciate how another person maybe thinking or feeling.

Endorphin. One of a class of neurotransmitters that can bind to the same receptors as opiates, such as morphine, bind to and produce the same effects of pain relief, euphoria and sleep.

Gate control theory. A theory of pain suggesting a functional gate in the spinal cord that either lets pain impulses travel onward to the brain or blocks their progress.

General adaptation syndrome (GAS). A consistent and general pattern of responses triggered by the effort to adapt to any stressor. The syndrome consists of three stages: alarm, resistance and exhaustion.

Generalised anxiety disorder (GAD). A condition that involves relatively mild but long lasting anxiety that is not focused on a particular object or situation.

Hippocampus. A structure in the forebrain associated with the formation of new memories.

Homeostasis. The tendency for organisms to keep their physiological systems at a steady, stable level by constantly adjusting themselves in response to change.

Hypnosis. An altered state of consciousness brought on by special induction techniques and characterised by varying degrees of responsiveness to suggestions for changes in experience and behaviour.

Hypochondriasis. A fear of physical illness without organic basis.

Hypothalamus. A structure in the forebrain that regulates hunger, thirst and sex drives. It has many connections to and from the ANS and to other parts of the brain.

Learned helplessness. A phenomenon that occurs when a person believes that they have no control over their environment. This may result in depression.

Limbic system. A set of brain structures that play an important role in regulating emotion and memory. The components of the limbic system interconnect with many other structures and influence numerous related functions.

Midbrain. Relays information from the sense organs and controls certain automatic functions. Nuclei in the midbrain are rich in endorphins and enkephalins and play an important role in pain modulation.

Neuromodulator. A neurotransmitter that in some circumstances modifies the response to other neurotransmitters at a synapse.

Neurotransmitter. A chemical that assists in the transfer of signals from the presynaptic cell to the postsynaptic cell.

Obsessive-compulsive disorder. An anxiety disorder in which a person becomes obsessed with certain thoughts or images or feels a compulsion to engage in certain repetitive behaviours.

Opioids. A class of neurotransmitters, including endorphins and enkephalins that are implicated in pain relief.

Periaqueductal and periventricular grey. Areas of the midbrain which are rich in opioids. These areas are involved in the descending inhibitory control of pain.

Peripheral nervous system. This comprises the somatic nervous system and the autonomic nervous system.

Personality. A pattern of psychological and behavioural characteristics unique to the individual.

Placebo. A physical or psychological treatment that contains no active component but produces effects because of the expectations and beliefs of the person receiving it.

Progressive relaxation. A procedure for learning to relax that involves tensing and releasing tension systematically in groups of muscles and focusing on the feeling of relaxation.

Psychoactive drug. A chemical substance that acts on the brain to produce a psychological effect.

Psychophysiological model. These models consider the interaction of physiological and psychological factors in the development of pain.

Psychophysiological studies examine the influence of mental events on physical changes which produce pain.

Psychotherapy. The treatment of psychological dysfunction through psychodynamic methods of analysing problems, providing support and encouraging more adaptive cognitions and behaviours.

Reinforcer. A stimulus event that increases the probability that the response that immediately preceded it will occur again. A reinforcer may be either positive or negative.

Reliability. The degree to which a test can be repeated with the same results.

Reticular formation. A network of nuclei and fibres throughout the brain which affects the activity of the rest of the brain.

Self efficacy. Ability to cope with a problem.

Somatic nervous system. The subsystem of the peripheral nervous system that transmits information from the senses to the CNS and carries signals from the CNS to the motor system.

Somatisation disorder. A disorder in which the person has numerous physical complaints without organic basis.

Substantaia gelatinosa. An area in Lamina II of the spinal cord where modulation or 'gating' of pain is theorised to take place.

Substantia nigra. An area of the midbrain involved in the smooth initiation of movement.

Thalamus. A structure in the forebrain that acts as a relay system and processing area for sensory information.

Type A personality. A personality type characterised by workaholism, intense competitiveness, aggressiveness, impatience and need for control.

Validity. The degree to which a test measures what it is supposed to measure.

Index

Page numbers in *italics* refer to figures and tables